WHAT THE HELL HAPPENED TO MY BRAIN?

of related interest

People with Dementia Speak Out
Lucy Whitman
Afterword by Professor Graham Stokes
ISBN 978 1 84905 270 2
eISBN 978 0 85700 552 6

Living Better with Dementia
Good Practice and Innovation for the Future
Shibley Rahman
Forewords by Kate Swaffer, Chris Roberts and Beth Britton
ISBN 978 1 84905 600 7
eISBN 978 1 78450 062 7

Intellectual Disability and Dementia
Research into Practice
Edited by Karen Watchman
ISBN 978 1 84905 422 5
eISBN 978 0 85700 796 4

WHAT THE HELL
HAPPENED TO
MY BRAIN?

Living Beyond Dementia

KATE SWAFFER

Forewords by Dr Richard Taylor,
Glenn Rees, AM and Dr Shibley Rahman

Jessica Kingsley *Publishers*
London and Philadelphia

First published in 2016
by Jessica Kingsley Publishers
73 Collier Street
London N1 9BE, UK
and
400 Market Street, Suite 400
Philadelphia, PA 19106, USA

www.jkp.com

Library of Congress Cataloging in Publication Data
Names: Swaffer, Kate, author.
Title: What the hell happened to my brain? : living beyond dementia / Kate
    Swaffer ; forewords by Glenn Rees, Shibley Rahman and Richard Taylor.
Description: London ; Philadelphia : Jessica Kingsley Publishers, 2016. |
    Includes bibliographical references and index.
Identifiers: LCCN 2015032755 | ISBN 9781849056083
Subjects: LCSH: Swaffer, Kate,--Mental health. |
    Dementia--Patients--Biography. | Alzheimer's disease--Patients--Biography.
    | Dementia--Patients--Care. | Dementia--Patients--Family relationships.
Classification: LCC RC523.3 .S93 2016 | DDC 616.8/30092--
dc23 LC record available at http://lccn.loc.gov/2015032755

British Library Cataloguing in Publication Data
A CIP catalogue record for this book is available from the British Library

ISBN 978 1 84905 608 3
eISBN 978 1 78450 073 3

Printed and bound in Great Britain

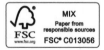

When it comes time to die, be not like those whose hearts are filled with the fear of death. Sing your death song, and die like a hero going home.

CHIEF AUPUMUT (1725), MOHICAN

Disclaimer

Information and other content included in this book is for general informational and educational purposes only and is not meant to be a substitute for the advice provided by a professional health care provider. You may not use or rely on any information contained in this book for diagnosing a health or medical problem or disease. You should always consult a professional health care provider regarding any health or medical condition, prevention, or treatment.

Do not delay or disregard seeking professional medical advice on account of something you have read in this book or on my websites www.kateswaffer.com and www.living beyonddementia.wordpress.com. Furthermore, comments made by others and approved for posting on my website are the opinions of the authors, and do not represent the opinions of Kate Swaffer.

Contents

Disclaimer		6
Foreword by Dr Richard Taylor		9
Foreword by Glenn Rees, AM		11
Foreword by Dr Shibley Rahman		13
Dedication		17
Acknowledgements		18
Author's Note		19
Introduction		21
1	Why Me, Why This, Why Now?	30
2	The Early Days	33
3	So, What the Hell Did Happen to My Brain?	37
4	Illness, Sadness and Positivity	51
5	The Dementia Train and Not Sweating the Small Stuff	54
6	Thank you, Richard Taylor	57
7	Reactions to Dementia: Yours, Mine, Others	60
8	The Burden of Disbelief	75
9	Being Diagnosed with Younger Onset Dementia	83
10	Children of People with Younger Onset Dementia	93
11	Early vs Delayed Diagnosis	103
12	Dementia, Grief and Loss: It's Very Complicated	109
13	The Emotional Toll of Letting Go	134
14	Myths of Dementia	139

15 Loneliness and Dementia   152

16 Prescribed Disengagement®   157

17 Dementia as a DisAbility   182

18 Stigma and Dementia   191

19 The Language of Dementia   197

20 Dementia and Word Finding   217

21 Employment and Dementia   219

22 Driving and Dementia   231

23 Family Care Partners or BUBs (Back-Up Brains)   239

24 Care Partners Speaking Out Publicly About
    People with Dementia   243

25 Guilt   250

26 Who's Got the 'Challenging Behaviours'?   259

27 Dementia and Common Sense   268

28 Interventions for Dementia   272

29 Blogging and Writing as Interventions for Dementia   284

30 Advocacy as an Intervention for Dementia   300

31 Volunteering as an Intervention for Dementia   308

32 Dementia-friendly/Accessible Communities   311

33 Human Rights in Dementia and Aged Care   331

34 There is Big Money in Dementia   340

35 Nothing About Us, Without Us…   344

36 Love, Gifts, Dementia and Dying   356

37 A Final Word on Resilience and Memory   359

38 Proof People with Dementia Can Live Beyond a
    Diagnosis of Dementia   364

    Dementia: A Brief Summary   *371*

    Resources   *382*

    References   *385*

Foreword by Dr Richard Taylor

Most folks I have met who are living with the symptoms of dementia (and I have spoken to and listened to hundreds and hundreds of them) begin their journey living with the symptoms of dementia following in the footsteps of the millions who have already heard the words 'You have dementia, probably of this or that type.' We focus on the very end stages of dementia. We tell ourselves, we act as if we have lost control of our lives, dreams, relationships. We begin to wait for the day our suffering ends and we will die, confused and alone. Personally, I cried for two weeks after I heard these words. Personally, I had no idea why I was crying. The stigmas of dementia incubate between the ears of most everyone walking the earth.

Kate Swaffer was no different from any one of us. What sets her apart, what makes it important that as many people as possible read this book, is her amazing insights to what, why, and how most of us are overwhelmed, frightened, confused, and afraid of our fate, once we have heard the diagnosis.

She brings a genuineness, an openness, an ethos which is comforting, informing, and deeply both positive and reassuring that we are okay. Our humanity is still and will always be intact. We all, still, and each have a future filled with opportunities for living a full and meaningful life. She not only practises what her book preaches, she lives it.

Kate brings a palpable sense of urgency to understanding and accepting those of us living with dementia and to the rest of her readers. It is an urgency that says stand up and speak out. Embrace your life. Do not become a victim of circumstances. To others (carers, professionals, friends and family) she asks, sometimes demands, they accept us as whole people.

If you want to know of a contemporary profile in courage, if you want to know dementia from the inside out – read this book.

Dr Richard Taylor
February 2015

Foreword by Glenn Rees, AM

No taboo is untouched in this book, whether it be suicide, euthanasia, loneliness or depression.

It is important that people without dementia understand the frustrations of a person with dementia after diagnosis. This book will challenge those who always know what is best for others – maybe all of us! It is a failing that makes a nonsense of person-centred approaches and giving reality to notions of choice in the decisions taken by the person with dementia and their families in the support and care that is needed.

This book underlines the importance of the slow recognition in Australia and across the world that dementia is as much a social as a medical condition. The unequivocal message is that as long as 'Prescribed Disengagement®' rules and the employment and other rights of those diagnosed are stripped away without thought, there can be no quality of life for those with dementia or their families. Being told to go away and get on with your life while removing the rights that others enjoy is not a treatment but a prescription for depression, frustration and anger.

We are treated in this book to the insights of a person with dementia that are not comfortable.

There is a transition in Kate's life from the time when she wrote 'My New World' for *Link Disability Magazine* when it was 'an effort not to just sit in a corner and cry' to the almost triumphant way she progresses to describing how she has taken up the challenge to take on the world, be herself and continue to achieve. In Kate's words, '…a diagnosis of younger onset dementia has finally given me real purpose and meaning, in the deepest sense of the word.'

Every person is unique and many will not have Kate's self-belief and courage in tackling her dementia head on.

There are issues which Kate and I will continue to dispute while remaining the best of colleagues. I think she is overly suspicious of dementia-friendly society approaches. There is of course a risk of simplistic approaches that do not address the fundamentals of cultural change. But it seems to me that unless we encourage all Australians to support the participation of people with dementia in society we will not get the changes in attitude that are so necessary. Centrelink, retail chains, banks and other businesses must provide access to services for people with dementia that all Australians have a right to expect.

Again I understand Kate's impatience with the need to move faster in being inclusive of people with dementia on advisory groups, Boards and the life of Alzheimer's organisations. But there has been a sea change since the turn of the century and some such as the Scottish Alzheimer's Society have blazed a trail long before others. I want to be positive because it is the only way to take others with us in achieving a better quality of life for people with dementia.

Glenn Rees, AM

Foreword by
Dr Shibley Rahman

First of all, I, too, would like to acknowledge the life of, and massive contribution made by, Richard Taylor PhD. Richard was a very wise man, remarkable in every way. His insights into his own experience of living with dementia are extremely important to us all.

Kate Swaffer, prior to this book, had already made a lasting impact in the academic field of dementia. Few people do. Her construct of 'Prescribed Disengagement®', through the analysis of 'disAbilities', provides a unique synthesis, and a fundamental resetting of the moral compass. Thanks to Kate's work, in large part, the direction of policy now is beginning to point away from simply drugs and towards helping people to get on with their lives. As Kate says, 'Dementia is the only terminal illness I know of where people are told to go home and give up, rather than to fight for their lives.' This, I completely agree, is unacceptable.

But now onto the book. This book is exceptional.

Although this book most clearly deserves to have a very wide readership, I think it should be carefully read by every clinician in training in every jurisdiction. Quite frankly, nobody else could have written this book. The author herself has excelled in a Master's degree in dementia care, having found meaning in her life with a diagnosis of young onset dementia.

What distinguishes this book is the fact that Kate is incredibly well-informed, and a personal determination shines through every word; and yet Kate writes with the beauty of poetry. The book is so well written, it actually does deserve the worn cliché that 'I couldn't put the book down.'

The narrative is way ahead of its time.

When Kate was diagnosed with dementia, the precise context was that the medical profession felt it could not do much. Such doctors typically earn their living through longitudinal follow-up of 'patients with dementia' to chart accurately the progression of 'deficits' and referring to other services where necessary. But this is entirely to miss the point, I now feel.

The critical issue is actually to support what a person can do, not what he or she cannot do. The medical profession is in a position of responsibility in not belittling its patients to a list of problems to be dealt with urgently often on a last minute basis. All citizens, whatever their precise status, should be interested in promoting wellbeing of persons living with dementia; this is to uphold a sense of mutual solidarity, justice, fairness, and dignity.

In wider world policy terms, this is no longer a question of being 'friendly', though I appreciate the sincerity and genuineness of this policy plank globally. This is, rather, about upholding rights, including in equality or human rights. Whilst this book is written in a 'dementia-friendly' style, I especially recommend this book to my colleagues in the health and care sectors. I certainly do not wish to undermine the terrific work being done in the search for symptomatic treatments, or possibly other medical interventions. But pumping resources into this endeavour should never be at the expense of the current generation of people who have received a diagnosis of a dementia. I suppose it's reassuring to use slogans and phrases such as 'keeping it real' or 'no decision about me without me', but I think we should all be on guard about promoting division inadvertently in this arm of policy.

This book will be invaluable to anyone who wishes to learn about aspects of living with dementia. I know of no other source which matches the quality and breadth of writing as in the book, in a brilliant and unique way; including young onset dementia, employment, the consequences of a delayed diagnosis, feelings of guilt, driving. And yet the book does not paralyse any subject through academic analysis. I recommend to you her unique chapter on blogging, for example. Kate's book, overall, therefore, takes the field of living well with dementia much further forward.

In fact, the book brings up topics that I really wish my academic colleagues had made much more progress on by now, such as tying up the grief and loss reactions to the effect of receiving a diagnosis of dementia. The book further broaches sensitive topics in a unique, incredible way so as not to make people feel uncomfortable; such as personal reactions about dying, or fears about the future.

One of the unfortunate fault-lines in the literature has been to assume in an uncritical way that people living with dementia necessarily should have the same agendas as caregivers. One of my favourite parts of the book is Kate's analysis of how care partners speak out publicly about people with dementia. Again, this is a topic people have been frightened to talk about.

I feel Kate through this book will ultimately reach out to millions, whether they are living with dementia or not. A word I have often heard used about Kate is 'inspirational'. In these days of hyperbole in the media, it is not uncommon for this word to be used, but in Kate's case it is richly deserved. Kate acts a focus for acknowledgement for values and attitudes which are right about this world, in generosity and warmth of spirit; of being educated, and great fun to be with. I know Kate's family means a lot to Kate, and I can only imagine how proud they must feel with this amazing book.

This book is highly original. I think it makes the weather on so many key topics, such as the abuse of language, or myths about dementia. Whilst it may make some people feel uncomfortable, including 'experts' and people in the media, they need not just to hear but to listen carefully. And the book somehow combines being timeless, placeless, and yet firmly relevant to us all, in the here and now, and clearly ahead of its time. But this inherent contradiction about the book does not particularly worry me, because of its sheer brilliance.

Sadly, I don't think this book will ever be matched in quality on the subject of dementia – unless of course Kate ever decides to do a follow-up.

I am honoured to now know Kate well as a close friend. She inspires me. She teaches me so much.

Dr Shibley Rahman
London
January 2015

Dedication

I dedicate this book to my brilliant and loving husband Peter who is my best friend who loves me unconditionally, and to my two amazing and talented sons Charles and Matthew. I love each one of you with every ounce of my being, and don't have enough words to thank you for your love and support, or to tell you how much I love you, or of the absolute joy you bring to my life.

We have shared our lives together with openness and honesty, and with laughter and the deepest love I have ever known. What more could this girl possibly want... Thank you.

Acknowledgements

Mr Glenn Rees, who was until late 2014 CEO of Alzheimer's Australia for 15 years and who is now the Chair of Alzheimer's Disease International (ADI), is one of the few professionals I know who truly has faith in people with dementia, and who never demeans or degrades us; he has always found ways to give us the chance to participate more fully. I imagine this has at times been against the tide in the organisation he worked for and quite possibly his Board, and even now at ADI. I will never really know, but I know without his belief in me, and his vision for all people with dementia, I would have given up, and globally, as a group, people with dementia would not be where they are today with what is becoming an increasingly powerful global voice. Thank you, Glenn.

Many continue to ask why I bother to write and blog, and speak out, and that remains relatively simple to answer, but without my husband, my two sons, Glenn Rees and a number of very special friends, I suspect I would have given up. Of course there are many others who cheer me on or inspire me, too many to list here, and also for fear of missing someone out, I have stopped at just a few. Suffice to say, I thank you all.

Author's Note

Some sections and sentences of the book may be repetitive – this is part of my disAbility and I have trouble seeing repetition as I cannot always remember what I've written or read. I hope not to be too repetitive throughout the book, but repeating things does help us retain information more easily, so perhaps, if I have been repetitive, we can simply call it being dementia-friendly!

This is a poem I wrote not long after diagnosis, which won second prize in competition at the University of South Australia. Thankfully I no longer feel as traumatised by or fearful of the diagnosis of dementia, and have learned to live beyond it, for now forgetting friends and family only occasionally. However, life as I once knew it, albeit still very slowly, is very quietly slipping away.

SLIPPING AWAY

Life slipping away
Terrified one day soon
I won't know my children

Life slipping away
Mortified one day soon
I won't know my husband

Life slipping away
Disbelief one day soon
I won't know my family

Life slipping away
Angry one day soon
I won't know my friends
Humiliated one day soon
I won't know how to drive

Life slipping away
Despairing one day soon
I won't know who I am

Introduction

Just like my first book of poetry, *Love, Life, Loss: A Roller-Coaster of Poetry* (2012c), this book is about my life, but with a particular focus on living with a diagnosis of younger onset dementia. It is not specifically an autobiography, but rather more about how I feel living with dementia, and of stories and thoughts from my heart, not only about dementia. It is not an academic book, nor specifically focused towards the health care sector; it is not a book only for people with dementia or their families or care partners. I do believe though that academics, health care professionals and service providers will learn from it too. It is written from the perspective of my truth, and my own reality. One could say the genre is confused, perhaps just like me some of the time. It is part creative non-fiction, part academic, and part autobiographical in style. Some stories or thoughts will resonate, some may not. Some may even annoy, but always, it will be from my heart.

I started writing about dementia to stay inspired, to share my thoughts, to remind me of *who I really am*, and to keep tabs on my life, my thoughts and my philosophies so that later on, I would have a record of them, even if I could not *remember* what I was thinking or doing. Through writing and blogging I have also been creating my own memory bank. The acquired habit of using social media such as Facebook and Twitter has also brought with it a discipline of making the effort to communicate, and in fact social media is almost the only way to connect with others these days as few answer their mobile phones, even fewer people answer their home phones if in fact they have one, and almost no-one has time for a coffee and a chat any more. It seems we are all too busy with our lives to talk to each other, and so writing is my way of staying connected, even if it is just in this book or through cyberspace on my blog or through social media. For now my blog, *Creating Life with Words: Inspiration, Love and Truth*,[1] and social media is often the only way I have of staying connected with myself and the rest of the world.

> *No-one picks up phones*
> *No time for idle chatter*
> *One short text will do*

Before writing and setting up my blog I hadn't realised how important it might be to create a shared space where other people with dementia and our families and friends could talk of life, illness, dementia and our other ever-deteriorating abilities, where I could discover in the witness of others (readers, rather than critics) how my stories had been heard. The insightful writer Joel Magarey, author of *Exposure*, felt his words had not been rendered alive until acknowledged by the reading and response of his soul mate and lover, whose compassion and timbre with him is described with such gracefulness in the book. He writes:

> As I imagine myself saying the words to Penny, they seem to gain the significance I want them to have as if only when I tell her of these solitary experiences will they come to truly exist. (2009, p.183)

1   http://kateswaffer.com

Such 'listening' reading requires philosophical and considerate silence allowing the author to speak to the imagination of the reader, and from the heart. It is not a substitute for more critical reading but can be a valuable source of human enrichment.

This book was born out of a lack of representation of people with dementia. I have read many books and blogs now, some of them deeply moving tributes to loved ones with dementia, educational, informative and offering support for care partners, but about people with dementia, by people without dementia. Sadly, I mostly find them, as well as many of the care partners' presentations I have seen online, highly distressing as so often the person with dementia is being written or spoken about in terms of how much of a burden they are to their family, and how we have 'faded away' or are 'not all there', which exacerbates the vast number of myths and stigma that go against the flow of living beyond dementia, and increases my guilt for having dementia.

I regularly feel exasperated that people without dementia continue to think it is okay to lecture, write, speak and present on what it is like for people with dementia, and what is best for us, and for much of the time without ever bothering to ask us. I am no longer willing to attend a conference or event about dementia if there is no-one with dementia on the podium as an invited keynote speaker.

I speak out because the phrase 'nothing about us, without us' has been bantered globally in the dementia sector for many years, and before that for many years in the disAbility sector, and yet full inclusion has not yet occurred. The World Dementia Council has been in existence since early 2014, and before a significant amount of advocacy for inclusion, no-one with dementia was a member. Every advocacy organisation in Australia, and most other countries' Alzheimer's associations or societies, whose vision statements say they are advocating for and supporting people with dementia and family care partners, rarely have people with dementia on their Boards. I believe it is a gross oversight, and simply supports the fact it is still more often about us, but without us. White Papers and other reports are missing the voices of people with dementia. It is not only insulting and offensive, it is discriminating, and continues to stigmatise, isolate and exclude us. Some might wonder why we would want to be on a Board anyway, as they can be tiresome and hard work, but by being about us, without us they continue to exacerbate the myths of dementia. I also speak out to educate others and raise awareness that dementia can happen to anyone, at any age. On top of that, if I don't invite you into my world, how can I reasonably expect you to understand what living with dementia is really like for me?

The other reason I decided to write and speak out about what it is like living with dementia – from the diagnosed person's point of view – is that I am tired of hearing and reading how much of a 'burden' we are to family care partners, how hard it is for them, how we are fading away, how our 'challenging behaviours' negatively impact them, and about how difficult the health care system finds caring for us in general. I am tired of listening to or reading articles from people without dementia, telling me how it is absolutely their right to lock people with dementia up or electronically track us. The rider of course is always that it is for our own safety.

When did it become legal to lock people up or electronically track them (for what others perceive is for our own safety)? As far as I know, only when we have been convicted as a criminal. Even people with severe mental illness cannot simply be locked away, and yet, society is still glibly accepting it is okay to continue to breach basic human rights by locking people with dementia away, or electronically tracking us. We place people with dementia into institutions, often secure dementia units and many often then forget about them. That is not just my opinion, as research clearly indicates that once a person has been admitted into residential aged care, they get very few visitors. It is sometimes simply not in the interest of the person going into residential care. Of course, this is a generalisation, although supported by research, and there are many family care partners who spend a lot of their time with the person they love, and who felt they had no choice but to place them into residential care. I was one of them, having been a family care partner for three people who had dementia, all now deceased. It is also important here to mention the guilt many family care partners feel after placing someone they love into residential care. Personally, my husband and I will probably always feel guilty, and that we failed his father, for having done so.

However, it is also worth pondering on the fact that we stopped locking children up in institutions many years ago, because we knew the care received in an institution was often poor and led to abuse. Yet we are still placing our elderly and people with dementia into institutions, ignoring these facts, and claiming it is 'for their own good'. Short rant over... More in Chapter 33 on human rights, a rather contentious subject when applied to the current status quo of aged and dementia care.

Since being diagnosed with dementia, I have become committed to providing an environment and forum for a meaningful dialogue with a wide range of stakeholders about the critical issues impacting a person living with a diagnosis of dementia. I am also striving to be motivated and positive, as well as remaining loving, adventurous, and serious when I need to be. Always, I try to be courteous, conscientious, courageous, thoughtful, honest, fun-loving, and attentive to detail, as well as focused on living a good life, wearing clean shoes and using my manners. I listened to an interview of Tony Bennett, one of my favourite singers, a few years ago, and when he was asked how he would like to be remembered, he replied, 'I want to be remembered as a nice person.' I too aspire to this simple yet profound philosophy. As you can see, I am rather an old-fashioned girl, somehow managing to survive the 21st century.

We live until we die. For the most part, I try to live as well and as positively as possible, to enjoy the days I am alive, always seeking to view my world as one with a glass half full.

Writing a book had been an idea of mine for the last few years, and in some ways was already very much in progress prior to being contacted by my publisher. However, I had not become organised enough to start contacting publishers myself. When I was contacted about whether I had thought of writing a book via Twitter, it was the inspiration I needed to finish writing this book, and has inspired me with a second and third book to follow this one, both already in progress. This book is not a piece of academic writing, but more a collection of personal stories and thoughts from my heart and soul, with some parts of it written in an academic style where I felt it necessary to illuminate a topic further.

The major challenge I have found writing this book is less about the disAbilities of dementia that I live with, and more about the emotional toll of re-living every single moment of my life before and especially since diagnosis.

My darling husband said he could never write about it… way too sad. So, as I am writing and editing, living inside the denial bubble is impossible, and many of the feelings of grief and trauma have been reopened. Nevertheless, it is very important that the voices of more people with dementia speak out on how they (we) feel living with dementia, and on what they think is best for them. Although this collection of personal stories and ideas is not only about my experience of living with dementia, that is the main theme, and I hope might pass the baton on to inspire others living with dementia to share their own stories and to speak up for what is best for them as individuals.

My life has been full of loss and grief, and Chapter 12 on that topic is longer than many of the others, because I believe the topic of grief and dementia has not been adequately explored in the literature, and is not sufficiently a part of our post-diagnosis dementia support.

When my father-in-law was diagnosed with Lewy body dementia and eventually ended up in residential aged care, I too had been diagnosed, and when I was volunteering in the coffee shop there, the other volunteers used to jokingly say, 'Here comes the demented, here to look after the demented!' Although I rail against the use of the word 'demented' because I find it completely offensive and disrespectful, in the same way I would be offended by being called retarded, in this particular environment I forgave them as it was said at the time with love and laughter. I will, however, discuss more on the language of dementia in Chapter 19.

Bob De Marco wrote about sharing stories on his website, The Alzheimer's Reading Room:

> Sharing allows each of us to unleash the inherent goodness that we each possess. By sharing little pieces of ourselves

we improve the lives of members of the Alzheimer's and dementia community around the world.[2]

I hope through my expert lived experience of living beyond a diagnosis of dementia, and by talking about some of my experiences, the good, the bad and the downright ugly ones, both prior to and since diagnosis, it will help you to understand what it is really like for those of us who are diagnosed and living with a dementia.

My other dream for this book is that it will help to create change and bring new insights to the dementia sector in general, and to service providers, medical practitioners, nurses and paid care partners, researchers and the community in general, as well as those diagnosed, and those people supporting us, as change is desperately needed. If it does this, then it will have exceeded all of my expectations.

My goal for this book is also to be thoughtful and honest, as well as provocative, as I do not believe dementia care is being done well as the norm, nor are we treated or respected as whole human beings by some in the sector, or the community as a whole. I would say, though, that in the last few months, in my travels in Australia and overseas, I sense a change, and professionals and researchers are really starting to listen and to want to make positive changes. It is very encouraging, and the relief I feel is sometimes palpable.

A dear friend of mine, Judy, who has been living with Alzheimer's disease for more than ten years and who has been advocating for the voices of people with dementia, has lived alone as long as I have known her. She was an inaugural member of the Alzheimer's Australia Dementia Advisory Committee (AADAC), and although now retired from that position remains a dear friend. I wanted to include

---

2   www.alzheimersreadingroom.com/2012/12/sharing.html

a whole chapter written by her about the challenges of living alone, but due to space constraints have been unable to do so. Although I know there are many great challenges for this particular group, I also wanted to say that from my outside view of those people with dementia who live alone, in some ways, perhaps because they have to work harder to support themselves, they appear to be doing better than many of those who live with a partner. They are not disAbled or disempowered by someone trying to support them.

There are also many voices missing in this book. The voices of the LGBTIQ, Aboriginal, homeless, intellectually disAbled, Indigenous, culturally and linguistically diverse (CALD), as well as those living alone are missing, and although I have included a little on the voices of the children and older parents of people with young onset dementia, these two groups deserve so much more. I have not had the space to include all voices here, but hope in future publications to cover more of them in more detail.

Since I began writing and then speaking and presenting in public, I have become part of a global movement of the authentic voice of people with dementia, by people with dementia, and I encourage more people with dementia to start speaking up.

If you don't, someone else will, and what others decide is best for you or me, may not be what we want. At last, at least here, it is no longer 'about us without us'.

> *To be nobody but yourself*
> *in a world which is doing its best,*
> *Night and day,*
> *to make you just like everybody else,*
> *Means to fight the greatest battle*
> *there is to fight,*
> *and never stop fighting.*

(E.E. CUMMINGS)

CHAPTER 1

Why Me, Why This, Why Now?

My soul was yearning
For days gone by of freedom
Lost to dementia

(KATE SWAFFER 2012)

There are many times I have wondered: *Why me, why this, why now?* This is the question everyone probably asks themselves when they are diagnosed with dementia, or in fact any other terminal illness or chronic condition, or when going through a life crisis such as a divorce or the death of a loved one. It is part of the grief process, as we come to terms with 'bad' news.

Dementia is not well understood in our community, and mostly considered an old person's disease. It is often also thought to be a mental illness, which it is not. This book has evolved from a desire to change attitudes and disrupt this type of myth, and break down issues such as the discrimination and stigma surrounding dementia. I am also hopeful it will help to improve the services for, and service provision provided by the whole health care sector to, people diagnosed with this insidious disease.

Soon after being diagnosed, the first formal writing I did about the experience was done for a subject at the

University of South Australia. It was meant to be a travel piece, as if I was a travel writer, about visiting a new place. The only 'place' I had inside my head was Mr Dementia, and with permission I wrote about that instead. It was subsequently published in the *Link Disability Magazine*. This is part of what I wrote:

> Dementia is an uninvited visitor to my world, an unwelcome early 50th birthday present, one where the old me seems to be rapidly moving away from a new me. I am being dragged along on this journey with no way to get back home as it races along like an express train without brakes. I read then I forget; I read, I take notes, and then I forget; I read, I highlight and take notes, and I still forget. That photographic memory I once had is gone, dead and fully buried. My high functioning mind has slipped away, sometimes showing itself like a ghost, teasing me into believing it will be okay, but just outside of my reach. Words now have no meaning and whole patches of my memory are disappearing.
>
> The mountain I am climbing is finite, but even if I get to the top there will be no grand planting of my flag nor will I have remembered the climb, and when I come down, I won't remember having been there. Some of my friends inform me I am not aphasic, that I am not remembering any less well than they do, that their world is the same as mine. They say I am getting old and this is what it is like, so get used to it. I ask myself, 'What would they know?'
>
> They are wrong. It is different. I regularly do not understand or remember what I read, or what people say to me... Reading has become a pointless exercise, due to the fact that as I read one paragraph, I have already forgotten the last. So taking notes of every single thing I read that I will need to recall has not become an option. Even writing a simple email or card to a friend has become a major task, because if I don't go slowly, or take the time to edit it over

and over, the words come out wrong. Writing is also difficult, as I can forget what I've written, and what the words mean.

It is insidiously depriving me of a normal existence, and is very humiliating and awkward to live with, stealing my soul, and threatening my very existence. It makes me nervous to go out. Every day now feels like a brand new one, except that my body feels very old and tired. I realise that not writing about my dementia is not an option and that no matter how long it takes to make it legible and worthwhile to read, it is important to the management of this disease. It is possibly the only form of therapy that will ease my stress and tears...

Most days are now an effort not to just sit in a corner and cry, not to just give up or to give in to it. It requires a great amount of emotional effort to live a 'normal' existence and is the most demeaning and frightening experience I have had, with a feeling of wretchedness I have not felt before.

This new place is full of hidden and impending madness, full of people already whispering behind closed doors away from my ears, trying to plan for my demise and how I and they will cope. They provide words of comfort and gentle pats on my back, meaning well but never realising it usually makes me feel as like a leper, as if I am to be pitied. They are the ones who will eventually have the challenges of coping, as I will be lost in a world of inhibition and supposed joyfulness, locked out of the reality of the world and its occupants. And so, I keep asking myself am I to be the lucky one in this strange place called dementia. Perhaps so! (Swaffer 2008)

To say the diagnosis of younger onset dementia was a shock is the understatement of the century! Initially it was all I could think about, and the profound grief almost consumed me.

CHAPTER 2

The Early Days

I was born in 1958 in a small country hospital at Cleve, and grew up in a farming community on South Australia's Eyre Peninsula on a property with approximately 5000 acres of mixed farming, and attended Cleve Area School. I was raised in an old-fashioned family, both parents having been raised in strict vaguely fundamentalist Christian families, and where studying and having a career was not encouraged for girls. An unusual attitude considering it was the 1970s, but one that had subconsciously been drummed into me from birth. It was done with the best of intentions, but definitely out of line with the changing times for women.

Studying was my love, and in the early days at school I preferred to spend more time in the library during lunch breaks than in the playground, although as the need to 'fit in' strengthened, more play and less study took place (and, as I was reminded at a fortieth school reunion in 2014, especially when an interest in the opposite sex reared its very distracting and youthful head! One thing I'll always ponder is why young people develop all those hormones and pheromones at exactly the time it is more important to work on getting through school and university and finding employment).

Nursing almost certainly became an escape option, one where I could earn a living, as well as have a career and accommodation in the nurse's quarters. It was definitely not my first choice, but was a meaningful and enjoyable career and one in which I had marvellous fun along the way.

I'd mucked around with many careers, almost as if by accident, and ironically had loved all of them, although as mentioned I am a glass half-full kind of girl. I have worked as a nurse in operating theatres, and as a chef in my own hospitality business. But they were not remotely in the same basket as my childhood dreams. Being a vet, a surgeon or a physiotherapist all comes to mind and I toyed with the idea of law in my late twenties, even studying it for a year. I had also dreamed of being a hostess in a function centre, and a writer, so to say I was stuck on one thing would be untrue! Even now, there are things I still want to do, some probably not yet thought of!

As a mother of a young child and after a difficult divorce I decided to give up my nursing career, and changed to wearing a chef's hat, which I did for almost ten years, running three successful and separate businesses under the umbrella of my company, Babette's Feasts Pty Ltd, named after one of my favourite 'foodie' movies, *Babette's Feast*. This new career started with *Kate Swaffer's Katering*, and after two years I purchased a wholesale cake business called *Café Cake*, and moved my businesses into a heritage listed function centre set on 4.5 acres called Beaumont House in the eastern suburbs of Adelaide. From there I ran corporate and private functions including weddings, my cake business and my corporate and private catering. For other serious health reasons, I gave up these businesses and quite by chance some time later, after my health returned, I was asked to apply for a position working as an executive in health care sales.

Volunteering has always been a big part of my life. After losing a partner, David, to suicide at the age of 27, I became involved in a suicide grief support group, and was Chairman and a volunteer grief support worker for the Bereaved Through Suicide Support Group Inc. for over nine years. I am still involved with them on a Professional Advisory Board. I'm also involved as a volunteer with The Big Issue in South Australia, an organisation supporting the homeless whose motto is *a hand up not a hand out*, which I love. There seems to be little use feeding people without also teaching them how to fish.

In my early thirties, becoming a psychologist was high on my agenda. Still, I didn't get around to it. I was working, I had remarried, we were bringing up children, and in retrospect life was a bit of a blur. Not in a bad way at all, but for any of you who have had school-age children, and worked full time, as well as either been a single parent, been through a divorce, owned and run a business, or all three, and then having a new husband who worked more than he was at home, you'll know what I mean. There simply was not any time to pursue any of my personal dreams, or any spare cash left over for them after paying for private school fees.

When diagnosed with a younger onset dementia I was in the prime of my life, and in many ways making up for lost time. Studying at university, the dreams of my youth, was like my recreational hobby, and for me much more fun than knitting, although likening it to knitting is how I had to explain it to my father to stop him nagging me to stop studying. I was working as an executive in health care sales, studying a double degree, caring for our school-age children and running our home with my husband, as well as volunteering in a nursing home and in the children's schools doing tuck shop, reading and fundraising. My life was (and still is) interesting, busy and very fulfilling.

I was (and cheerfully still am) happily married with two sons, who were 16 and 17 at the time of my diagnosis, the youngest at that time in year 12 at school. My two sons Charles and Matthew were and still are my main priority and along with Peter, my husband now of 17 years, they are the greatest loves of my life. Of course, the boys might dispute this, and say it is my cat, and for anyone who reads this and also follows me on Facebook or Twitter, you might actually agree with them!

So there I was, almost a million good and bad experiences later, happily married for the third time, working full time, loving life, studying a double degree, and hoping to go on to become either a crime writer or a Clinical Psychologist! I'd 'survived' a number of other serious illnesses, an ugly divorce, a loved one's death through suicide, domestic violence, entrapment, and a whole range of other unpleasant things, but I was still living life to the max and starting to actually do some things for me when I was diagnosed with a younger onset dementia at the age of 49, probably semantic.

CHAPTER 3

So, What the Hell Did Happen to My Brain?

STOLEN DREAMS

stolen dreams smashed against a brick wall
disappearing into nothingness
feeling cheated angry deeply sad
the six words that created my new world
what bad luck you have dementia
This train is racing down a one way lane
no chance to get off no chance of anyone getting on
never to return to the place I once knew
tears escaping from swollen eyes down blotchy cheeks
the taste of salt a permanent flavour
my soul mate angry and crying both feeling cheated
we were two sides of the same coin
knowing each other intimately and completely
best mates and passionately in love
aware of each other's thoughts before they were spoken
conscious of each other's inner worlds sadness or joy
our new world is collapsing into one of fear and
*   trepidation*
somehow we must find the good in yet another crisis
our love will get us through it has before
but the effort will be gigantic

the world at the other end is
too scary to think about
he said he will hate it when I forget who he is
then he said with a sense of despair
please don't call me by your ex-husband's name
and at this we laughed out loud
even though the gravity of this new world
hit us between the eyes like a piercing hot needle

(KATE SWAFFER 2008)

This chapter is about what it was like in the early days before and after diagnosis.

The title of this book is based on the niggling question I have had since well before my formal diagnosis. I had a photographic memory in many areas, for example I could remember phone numbers, addresses, postcodes, bank account and credit card numbers of all members of my immediate family, and if I concentrated, and used two senses at the same time when learning new information, I remembered it. This was fabulous in particular for things like examinations at school and nursing, but unsettling when it noticeably changed.

In 2006, I started spelling that wrong (taht) and becoming confused about the use of words like *there* and *their*, and then other very simple word mistakes. These things possibly started as far back as my early forties, as I found recorded in one of my notebooks that I was getting the colours purple and orange confused, and then red and green back to front, which obviously made it challenging to drive as I started stopping suddenly at green traffic lights and running through red lights. Number sets were getting confused, for example seeing 9 as 8, and I was seeing words in strange ways, for example words like castle suddenly started appearing to me as two words, 'cast' and 'lee'. I had been exceptional at language, and losing these skills was confusing and eventually moderately concerning.

Then in 2007 I needed people at work to start checking my quotes, reports and letters. This seemed odd to them, and increasingly distressing to me.

Having come from a high intellectual base, which is not meant to sound egotistical, but rather to put things in real perspective, when I discovered signs of dyslexia, memory loss (more than just what I knew to be the benign senescent memory loss normal for my age) and significant challenges in my ability to process simple information, I started to think something was wrong.

With increasing features prominent to dementia including impaired cognition and comprehension, mild speech difficulties and language dysfunction, increasing episodic memory loss, mild anomia, and surface dyslexia, I was first formally examined in 2007.

When I was sent for my first MRI (magnetic resonance imaging) scan, I was not even insightful enough to have realised I was being checked for Alzheimer's disease. This was one significant alert to my neurologist, as I had been a nurse, and once would have been very aware of what and why medical tests were being performed on me.

The first batch of neuropsychology tests showed my memory was just below average for someone my age, which was truly devastating, but treated very glibly. Coming from a high IQ, it was devastating to be told I was 'just below average for my age', and many times I was spoken to as if I was just a person with an average intelligence, with imaginary symptoms or perhaps 'suffering from depression', rather than a *real* disease. I had then, and still have, no problems with being told I have depression, in fact would prefer it to dementia as it is not terminal and is treatable, even though the stigma is probably still about the same.

Compensation for these disAbilities was initially very easy, but in 2008 further brain scans and neuropsychology tests were performed which showed increased deficits in the semantic categories, increased anomia, object and auditory agnosia, increased surface dyslexia, and prosody, which is the inability to understand poetry, quite significant at the time as I had been studying poetry and although I could write it, could not understand it. I also had mild behavioural changes and my number cognition was impaired.

After further decline, and further humiliating and invasive tests, the diagnosis was made, followed up with a second neurologist and neuropsychologist interstate at the Box Hill Memory Clinic who re-confirmed the diagnosis in 2009. The affected areas at the time were my left temporal and right and left parietal lobes, but predominantly the left temporal lobe.

The only way to know 100 per cent that someone has dementia is with a brain biopsy (autopsy), which I'm not quite ready for!

Again, to say it has been a roller-coaster ride is an understatement! My life has changed in ways that are challenging to understand and live with, and yet somehow I manage to use these things to strengthen my resilience and drive to achieve more of my goals…to live every day as if it is my last, just in case it is, and I urge you all to 'live with urgency, before the emergency' (Moore 2011).

In 2011 I wrote an article published in *The Big Issue* and this is part of what I said back then.

My high functioning mind has slipped away, sometimes showing itself like a ghost, trying to tease me into believing it will be okay, but now outside of my reach. My thoughts fly around inside my head like helium balloons high inside an auditorium, also out of my reach. (Swaffer 2011a)

I do still wonder, on the bad days, 'What the hell happened to my brain?'

The feeling that my life is slipping away from me is almost tangible. It is more certain and I sense stronger than before and I do sometimes feel cheated. Losing my legs and arms or my sight or hearing, or even contracting AIDS might be better than this hideous disease. When I was first diagnosed, the tears ran down my cheeks, non-stop for almost three weeks. The only solace then was I occasionally would forget why I'd been crying. I used to think 'if only someone would tell me it is just depression or some bizarre mental illness…anything other than dementia'.

Being told I had dementia was like a pseudo-death! I was not to know that this experience of loss would be repeated over and over again; not one person or book warned me of that fact, and in the chapter on grief I hope to cover that in more detail.

Just as sudden as the death of a loved one, but of parts of me! I have been told that my telling of my story has special significance for others. My blog is full of stories and thoughts, frank and open, giving some insight into the ups and downs from the diagnosed person's perspective. Havi Carel would call this the first-person experience, and she also cites Epicurus' and Heidegger's ideas of death, both of them ultimately 'unifying the first-person existential perspective with the third-person perspective of philosophy' (2008, p.116).

It is more than that for me; it is the means by which I heal my soul, allowing my mind and body to keep striving for wellness, excellence and peace. The hard drive I had is slowly evaporating as I remember a face, but often cannot

remember a name, or as I search for a 'thing', the name
of which I cannot remember, making my language more
generic. The lapses of memory are intermittent, not all the
time, sometimes short-term, sometimes long-term memories
are affected. On the good days it tempts me into believing
nothing is wrong when it seems perhaps it is only a memory
loss that is normal at my age. The multi-tasking I was so
good at has gone, and sometimes I can barely manage one
function, getting distracted part way through completing a
simple task, then forgetting what I had been doing.

My house consists of laminated signs on cupboards and
walls now, hopefully helping me to get dressed on the days
I find it a struggle or, more importantly, to not burn down
the house as I now leave the gas burners on too often for
comfort. I use Webster packs to manage medication, with
electronic reminders in my calendars and on my phone,
and on my husband's phone as a back-up to check I have
taken it.

Having to accept extra supports like this feels humiliating
and frustrating, but the alternatives are worse, and so I have
had to get used to relying on support and others. I've come
to call things like laminated reminder sheets and a walking
stick my 'Life enhancement aids', and although annoying, I
have never hesitated or felt embarrassed to use my reading
glasses, so have encouraged myself to stop worrying about
any other aids.

The one message I really want anyone who reads this
book to get is the slogan from a group I am co-founder
of, Dementia Alliance International:[1] *See the person, not the
dementia.*

---

1   www.dementiaallianceinternational.org

In 2011 I wrote a blog called 'I miss my memory', and said it is hard to take, and that it needs to be. One of my blog followers has said:

> I have [been] trying to imagine what it must be like. We are all forgetful. Yet we can't actually force ourselves to forget. So I still have those memories of embarrassing moments of doing, saying the most stupid, awkward and sometimes for other [sic] hilarious moments!
>
> But forgetfulness is very different, it isn't permanent, that context still remains and often reignites the forgotten.
>
> But I get the impression that for you Kate these memories once forgotten are often gone forever? Have I understood you correctly? It is unimaginable! How scary it must be to be uncontrollably lost in a familiar place, your home town! Yet, on the hand, you write so well, so movingly. I feel your anguish.[2]

It may sound odd, but I miss knowing the names of most of the bones, muscles, organs and systems in my body and the diseases that may afflict you or me (I was once a nurse so would have known them). I miss the names of composers and symphonies, the names of songs and singers. I miss knowing all the ways to cook potatoes and cakes, how to use my hair dryer, knowing what order to put my shoes and socks on, and a million other things and moments in time. Sitting at a restaurant table, wondering if we have eaten, when in fact we are waiting for the bill; I will either get slim or very fat! Some days I mix up the hairspray and deodorant, ending up with sticky armpits and funny smelling hair!

My memory loss is random; some parts of the pencil drawing are still there, and other parts have disappeared. I can remember some parts of the puzzle, and have no

2   Comment posted to *Creating Life with Words* by Paul on 19 December 2011: http://kateswaffer.com/discussion-forum/#comment-330.

recollection of others. I have no idea why I cannot remember it, but I do know I miss remembering my girlfriend's wedding, and find it mystifying that I can remember her father's funeral, a few weeks before that.

I miss knowing if I have taken my medication today. I miss remembering if I have kissed my children or husband today or yesterday, or told them I love them. Some of the time, my written words, a conversation with someone or some other trigger can reignite the flame of a memory, and at other times it cannot; the landscape is sometimes desperately bare. There is no rhyme or reason, and this is also why it is easy on the good days for me, and others, to wonder sometimes if I really do have dementia. And then a 'bad' day appears.

I know in my heart the diagnosis is real but it has not been easy to come to terms with. Dementia used to feel as if my soul was being sucked out, little bit by little bit, and like watching myself slowly die. The Harry Potter wiki website describes Dementors like this:

> A Dementor is a Dark creature, considered one of the foulest to inhabit the world. Dementors feed off human happiness, and thus cause depression and despair to anyone near them. They can also consume a person's soul leaving their victims in a permanent vegetative state, and thus are often referred to as 'soul-sucking fiends' and are known to leave a person as an 'empty-shell'.[3]

For me, this confirmed how it felt, and sometimes still feels. In fact, the Dementors in the Harry Potter movies perfectly represent in a visual way how it feels having dementia, as if my soul is being sucked out. Although there are days it still

---

3   http://harrypotter.wikia.com/wiki/Dementor

feels like this, most of the time I am simply getting on with living in the best and most positive way possible.

Speaking and thinking is more difficult; the search for words, the meaning of words, numbers and equations are now a major challenge. I am seeing words in strange ways, not as whole words any more but as if they are split into two. The acquired dyslexia is changing terms like Hamish and Andy into Amish and Handy. It is much harder to hide the symptoms, or to rely on the inner voice I have been using to help me to think and to find the right words to speak. It is more difficult to process information, to know how to act and to respond, how to behave appropriately and to know what to do in normal everyday situations.

There are many more moments where the 'slips of my tongue or mind' are evident and my tongue twists as it struggles with the effort of finding the right words. Studying and writing has been greatly impacted, as it takes many more hours not only to understand what it is I am meant to do, but then to actually do it. For example it can take up to an hour to make a short email legible. My abilities are permanently damaged and my photographic memory is dead and buried!

Until my mid-forties, I had what I used to describe as at least 12 television screens running inside my head at the same time, and I was able to keep up with each separate story or activity as well as respond appropriately. There was a time in my life I held down a number of different paid jobs at the same time, including working night and day shifts in nursing, and never needed a diary. I operated like that for my whole life until the symptoms of dementia got in the way.

One thing my boys have said is since being diagnosed, they really miss me being the living telephone book! Once, if I heard it or read it, I remembered it. End of story.

Although uncommon in semantic dementia, hallucinations sometimes take over my mind, as strangers and wild cats occasionally stalk me. The feeling that these things are real is momentary, but startling none the less and they increase the feeling of madness creeping into my soul. I am hearing phones and doorbells ringing when they are not. I am becoming fixated on things, and adopting strange behaviours. There are times when I pour myself a glass of water, then drink from the bottle. It is no longer possible to be sure of what I will do or how I will perform, reducing my desire and enthusiasm to go out to socialise or to do simple things like shopping.

Money and how to manage it has become problematic. Managing the spreadsheets, BAS statements and the MYOB programme for our accountant is now not possible without help. I blow dry my hair less often as I sometimes cannot work out how to. I cannot always name a pair of socks. I am forgetting how to cook, even simple things like potatoes. This book, started some time ago, has taken years to complete.

The written word is now a lot easier than the spoken word, as thankfully my touch typing skills learned at high school have not disappeared yet. I only took the Typing and Shorthand class as an extra subject in second year high school because the teacher was the current Miss Australia; many of the boys that year did as well! There is, thankfully, also software such as spellcheck these days. However, I am increasingly struggling to find words, and with my speech, when I am too tired to paddle and these things have increased significantly as each year progresses, and my paddling has become much harder and more tiring.

You may ask, 'What do you mean by paddling?' The first time I heard it was in an episode of *The Inspector Lynley Murder Mysteries*, when Inspector Lynley talked about his mum possibly having Alzheimer's disease, and how she was like a swan paddling below the surface to stay afloat (function). Christine Bryden, a prominent Australian woman and herself living beyond dementia, also uses this analogy in her book *Dancing with Dementia* (2006, p.102). I can relate to this particular analogy, and have found as the years have progressed since diagnosis, my paddling is slowly becoming much more difficult.

As each day deals out a new challenge, a new loss, a renewed fear of what is happening to my brain, I fight to rise above it. I am getting used to what is unfolding in front of me, and now alarmingly unfolding in front of my close family and friends. It is trying to degrade my existence and it tempts me into feel less like a human being. One of the regular features of my life now is the fear of not remembering my close friends. Each time I meet with them, I walk away wondering will I recognise them the next time we meet. I still know that I know them, but now I often feel disconnected, as if I have been overseas for years, as many things they talk about seem new to me. I need the comfort of their reassurance and of being believed. There are also days when I don't remember them. As my new world evolves and the old one slowly disappears, the sense of trepidation grows.

It often feels as if I am drowning, with everyone looking on and me just out of reach, unable to be saved. The intensity of my fears and grief is hard to ignore as my world slowly disappears, a world which is spinning past me, taunting me to remember, to recognise it, teasing my mind in its capacity to function.

People often minimise our symptoms, or liken them to others, and in my case, especially people much older than me. The anticipation of the loss of my privacy and ability to care for myself is daunting. Knowing that my family and close friends will have to make decisions for my wellbeing, and that strangers may be managing my daily care and the way I am dressed, is more than uncomfortable. Feelings of humiliation and sadness, and the loss of my dignity regularly try to take over my daily thoughts.

The downward slide of this disease has brought with it an avalanche of responsibilities, fears and guilt. I continue to try to negotiate a secure footing with the ground relentlessly shifting beneath me.

There is no balance. There is no place of respite. Dementia can too easily represent the end of dreaming, a long and unforgiving one-way odyssey into obscurity, clouded in a thick and unforgiving fog; I prefer to strive to live beyond that.

I use non-pharmacological and positive psychosocial interventions to promote wellbeing and happiness, which I will discuss in more detail in Chapter 28. With no drug treatment options offered to me, and the realisation it is a terminal illness, I eventually accepted it as a disease with disAbilities to be managed, rather than symptoms contributing to my demise. Motor neurone disease (MND) was also placed on my table late in 2009, although it has not progressed at the expected 'rush towards death' suggested to me at the time, or was a misdiagnosis. Investigations have not completely ruled out the possibility that I have MND, and semantic dementia (SD) is often associated with motor neurone disease-type inclusions (Croot 2009), although for now I feel it must surely have been a misdiagnosis.

People with dementia have many losses, and sometimes it seems as if we are moving from one small death to another. Staying connected to family and friends, past and present is in many ways imperative to our health and happiness. Eventually, dementia can take that away, and so it is imperative that people with dementia are empowered to live beyond the diagnosis, at least while they still can, and not to give up instead.

Being diagnosed with dementia, and living with the symptoms of dementia, is definitely not as much fun as having a birthday party, but having dementia is no reason to give up living or to 'die' straight away. I continue to strive to live beyond dementia, as well as possible, and am in the greatest 'fight for my life' I have ever known. Whilst the language of war is not always helpful, it was the only phrase I could think of to describe the way I am living with dementia; I am, quite literally, fighting for my life, at least as much as I would if diagnosed with cancer.

These days I prefer to think of it as proactively doing everything possible to live beyond the diagnosis – not so much in spite of, but alongside dementia.

My life has been a constant quest for meaning, and I'm ecstatic to say, I think living with the symptoms of dementia, and a diagnosis of a younger onset dementia, has finally given me real purpose and meaning, in the deepest sense of the word.

Dementia pushed me to think about life without memories and with deteriorating functioning. It pushed me to live in the present, more than I ever had before.

The thought of not knowing what I have done or was thinking or saying is reasonably annoying; not being able to recall conversations is often more than a pest. Resilience and a positive attitude, something I was either born with or have developed through illness and adversity, has been the key to me living beyond dementia, and to finding strategies to see, and then actively support, the symptoms of dementia as disAbilities.

CHAPTER 4 ————————————————

Illness, Sadness and Positivity

Illness can illuminate your whole being with sadness, which can seem impossible to recover from. The stages of grief, ranging from anger and denial to the enveloping apathy and general lack of lust for life, take their toll on your ability to survive each day in the way the rest of the world expects you to. I believe that the lack of grief and loss counselling for people with dementia may be the cause of the high incidence of apathy and depression people with dementia experience, which I discuss further in Chapter 12.

In my search for the positives, I have not only found many things to be happy about, like being able to play cards alone, and always winning, but I have become more spiritually aware and it is my time to become truly enlightened, and for my family to face up to their own challenges as they come to terms with what is happening to me and to them. I have also become more acutely aware of the depth of beauty in the world, of the love I feel for my close family and friends, and of their love for me, and therefore of what we are all losing.

I have discovered I must learn to separate what is left of my mind from this illness, learn to live without restraint, free of the fear of dementia and death. I do not wish to be

51

herded into the human cattle yard for dementia otherwise known as the secure dementia respite care unit or a secure dementia ward in an aged care nursing home. I must focus my energy on what is good in life, as if there is nothing wrong with me, in order to have the energy to continue to pursue my goals and dreams, to spend good and happy times with my loved ones and to look beyond myself, beyond dementia, and to reach out to others in need and focus on helping them.

Pharmacological interventions are not available for my and for many other types of dementia, and due to this, and my proactive response, 'treatment' has been positive psychology and other non-pharmacological interventions. The advice of medical practitioners and some service providers was to give up work, give up studies and start living for the time I had left. This Prescribed Disengagement® (see Chapter 16) seemed at odds with what I perceived to be 'positive living', and so I eventually ignored it, instead developing strategies to be productive, setting up a regime of activities and lifestyle changes specifically focused on combating or supporting symptoms and increasing positive engagement.

Treating symptoms as the gateway to support for my disAbilities has become vital to my wellbeing and perceived longevity.

Illness has forced me to look inside my own heart, to accept my dark side, to delve into my own life deeply and to stop using my past as an excuse for not living life to the full. It has helped me to turn other negative experiences into inner strengths and to further develop my own resilience. It has helped me to embrace every new crisis wholeheartedly, to welcome them with open arms. Dementia and other illness is a large part of what has made me the person I am today. Mine is a life stained with pain, loss and sadness, but one that has offered the opportunity to seize life by the throat, and live without boundaries, forcing me to make a choice to survive, grow and heal rather than sit down and quietly die.

CHAPTER 5

The Dementia Train and Not Sweating the Small Stuff

THE DEMENTIA TRAIN

A lottery ticket
Lost inside an MRI machine

Results that reach into your soul
A pass for the dementia train
Slowly taking off

Speeding around corners
It stops at the station
But no way to get off

And no-one can get on
No fat controller here
Controlling the ride of my life
Taking me to nowhere

(SWAFFER 2012C, P.79)

My dementia train seems to stop for a while here and there, or at least to slow down, rumbling along the tracks slowly, rounding the bends with ease and going through the deep dark tunnels with the sense that the light at the end is still bright. It had once seemed to be stable, as if the dementia was not progressing. Well, not completely, but as if I would – or could – beat it. It seemed I could prevent the onslaught of those bloody Dementors, but they continue to suck away at my soul, making sure I have to work even harder to restore the ever-emptying shell.

Small events turn into mini-tsunamis; my mind will not always be able to regain proper perspective; nights awake wondering and worrying about conversations and events; paranoias and compulsions. Conversations full of promise and meaning, not fully remembered, or partially misunderstood, render my mind to mush, fill my soul with apprehension.

The dementia has definitely made life more complex, but has also unlocked new doors and interesting pathways, and found new mountains for me to climb and explore, albeit with more difficulty than before. I do believe I have slowed down the progression of the disease with the way I have learned to live with it, and in Chapter 28 I will talk about the many interventions I have been using.

My world has seemingly disappeared and expanded at the same time. I often ask myself: how can that be? Is it because of the way I choose to deal with the cards I have been dealt, or just the luck of the draw? Does this even matter? Apart from my family and close friends, who really cares anyway?

Not sweating the small stuff is so much harder when you have thoughts of fewer tomorrows sitting there, quietly colouring every moment. Worrying about the piece of fish on my plate being big enough, tasty enough, cooked enough, or whether I should have chosen chicken; surely I am just lucky enough to be able to eat out at all? Thinking about love, life, my family and those beautiful friends who have stuck with us on this train ride, and the fun we have together has to be, and is, enough.

There are currently more than 47.5 million others travelling this path of dementia (World Health Organization 2015), all with stories just as meaningful and painful as my own, each living with the same trepidation and emptiness, each facing the same fears and sadness, everyone trying in earnest to survive as well as they can. Being able to speak out is an honour and worth the effort if it helps enable and improve the care of those of us with this condition.

For now, my brain continues to allow me for much of the time to make sense of my world, to have some insight into what is happening to me and to my family, and because of this I feel I must speak out, especially for those with dementia who perhaps cannot, or who prefer not to publicly share their own experience of living with a dementia. Speaking out publicly is not for everyone, and there has certainly been quite a high emotional price to pay for having been a person who has chosen to do so.

It also helps me to make sense of this disease, to feel as if there is real value in this deck of cards.

Regardless of the effort I need to make to keep on top of this disease, there are still many days when I do not want to get out of bed, do not want to be bothered putting in the huge effort to get through the morning, let alone the day; for now I can still choose to soldier on.

It is important for me to spend the great times now, and I strive every moment of every day to develop a more welcoming approach to illness, disAbility, dementia and death. I try to see them as the gifts that they have become, and in some small way to leave this world a better place.

CHAPTER 6

Thank you, Richard Taylor

A hero is an ordinary individual who finds the strength to persevere and endure in spite of overwhelming obstacles.

(CHRISTOPHER REEVE)

The late Richard Taylor, PhD[1] was one of my heroes. His writings were the first I had discovered by a person living with dementia, and in many ways I feel his words 'saved my life'. By that, I mean he saved me from continuing down the very slippery slope of doom and gloom of dementia, the pathway the medical doctors, health care and service providers also send you upon diagnosis. I had not heard of anyone living well with or beyond dementia, and although referred to other books and writings, they did not suggest it was possible to live well with, or beyond, dementia. These other books, whilst somewhat helpful, did not really teach me I could live beyond dementia nor how to do that.

Richard Taylor taught me that, and my DisAbility Adviser Jayne Ayliffe[2] at the University of South Australia supported the idea. Mr Google had also become my friend.

---

1   www.richardtaylorphd.com
2   www.unisanet.unisa.edu.au/staff/homepage.asp?name=jayne.ayliffe

Richard Taylor definitely inspired me to rise above the downward spiral of Mr Dementia, and to learn to live beyond it and the following excerpt from one of his essays was the catalyst for me to start to write about my experience, and ultimately to find meaning on this wild ride.

Finding the right words

Is this the end of the beginning or the beginning of the end?

I am scared I am running out of usable time. Usable in the sense that I am using it now. I know I am not at the same level of general competency this January as I was last January. I am more dependent on others for assistance in performing the daily activities of living my current life. Clearly I could not keep this pace of activities without my spouse cleaning up behind me, reminding me to do this or that, asking if I wanted to do this or that. Taking care of me when I can't, and helping me to take care of myself when I need help. Her patience is both generous and essential.

I have good days and bad. Good hours and bad. Good moments and bad. There is no predicting when or how the bad ones will come, except when I am very tired. Sometimes I am aware I am floundering and cannot seem to hold myself together. It is strange watching yourself misdial a phone number, time after time after time. Look for a name and then forget what I was looking for right in the middle of my search. Stand up from my chair to do something and not have a clue as to what it was. Most dangerous for me are the moments I do not understand, but think I do, or do not remember. I say things, I tell people things, I think I understand situations that are not true, a little true, or from out in left field, and the worst part of it is I do not know when each of these moments are happening. Will I do something on this date? Sure. Except I wrote it on the wrong month in my calendar and did not find out for three weeks. Can I do this? Of course! When I really did not understand what was being asked of me, and I just said 'yes' for reasons that only Dr. Alzheimer knows.

Tie these all together; multiply them by 25 and you have an insight into my days. There is of course lots of time between the events, when I cruise along acting, and sometimes thinking like there is nothing wrong, until SPLASH – another glass of ice water in my face, compliments of Dr. Alzheimer. (Taylor 2008)

I had the great privilege to meet Richard in person a number of times, and feel incredibly honoured and proud to have been able to call him a close friend. He was also one of the co-founders of Dementia Alliance International, and a Board member for some time. He is still one of my mentors, even though he died on 25 July of this year from throat cancer. When we met for the first time in person in London in 2012 at the Alzheimer's Disease International (ADI) conference, my first time attending an ADI conference, he said he felt like we were kindred spirits. I felt the same then and even now still feel we are very spiritually and intellectually connected, regardless of the fact we can no longer speak in person or online. When he was diagnosed with throat cancer a couple of years ago, I grieved with and for him along with many other people who have found his influence and friendship important.

Dementia Alliance International held an online Memorial Tribute to honour Dr Richard Taylor, which you can access on their YouTube Channel.[3] It was more obvious after his death just how much impact he had and how many people who loved him and were inspired by him. Thank you, Richard Taylor.

3   https://www.youtube.com/watch?v=oxT1QWSqdQE

CHAPTER 7

Reactions to Dementia: Yours, Mine, Others

I sent the club a wire stating,
PLEASE ACCEPT MY RESIGNATION.
I DON'T WANT TO BELONG TO ANY CLUB
THAT WILL ACCEPT ME AS A MEMBER.

(GROUCHO MARX)

I feel that way about dementia, but as I have no choice, the
best way I can survive and live my life is to laugh often,
to ignore the negatives when I can, including the negative
reactions I get to having dementia, and to try to see the
good side of life.

(SWAFFER 2011)

When a person with dementia 'comes out' about their diagnosis, and openly admits they are living with the symptoms of, and a diagnosis of, a dementia, there are a number of reactions and responses. The person with dementia is thrown into complete turmoil; grief and often a lot of anger, and questions and suggestions such as; 'why me?', 'surely it can't be true', or 'let's get a second opinion'. There are many more feelings and reactions to getting a diagnosis of dementia. Not only for the person diagnosed but their family and friends. Coming to terms with such a diagnosis is a very difficult thing for every family facing the arrival of Mr Dementia, known in my household as Larry. This chapter hopes to explore some of them, specifically related to my and our own experience, but also observations of many other families who have the arrival of Mr Dementia in their lives.

I have said this previously, but the diagnosis of dementia really did feel like a pseudo-death, of me, and of who I am, my history, and then the fear of who I might become.

After being diagnosed and discussing it with my husband and sons, we decided the best thing to do was to 'come out' about it, and I use that phrase as it felt like what I imagine it might be like coming out if I had been gay. My apologies to anyone who is gay reading this, as it may not be like that at all, but it was my only way of describing it, the only analogy I could think of.

The first few weeks I cried non-stop, tears that felt as if they would never go away. Together, my husband and I walked almost every day for exercise and leisure, and some of those days, I started running, with salty tears running down my blotchy cheeks like river torrents. I cried and cried and cried, and thought they would never stop, but after you run long enough, the pain takes over and gives you something else to think about! It worked, at least when I was running.

Many days it felt like I was drowning (some days it still does) from the symptoms of dementia, and my husband and I often talk about the changes that are taking place, and the fear we both feel when I might not be able to keep myself afloat by paddling. It is not the most comfortable emotional journey, constantly feeling like I am being pulled under the current, swirling around almost out of control, people looking on but basically helpless to intervene. My husband feels helpless much of the time, and I know he also feels like he is failing me in not being able to 'fix' things. It is definitely a male trait to want to fix things, although I am very much like that too. The notion of drowning might be why I have previously titled my personal story *My Unseen Disappearing World,* as when you are drowning, you also disappear. It was also what I called my Adelaide Fringe performance in 2012, a few excerpts of which I will share later on.

Then finding those excerpts written by Richard Taylor almost saved my life.

I often refer to Richard as having saved my life, part of the reason I have a whole section devoted to him earlier in this book. Without writing about the emotional pain of being diagnosed with dementia, I also believe I would have developed depression. I've come close to being depressed a few times but, for now, always find writing and working hard on being positive helps me heal so that a clinical depression doesn't develop. I strongly recommend you try it, for any crisis or grief and loss, and especially if you are diagnosed with any sort of serious chronic or terminal illness.

I feel with some certainty that the depression many people with dementia are diagnosed with is more likely part of the grief we experience after the diagnosis, a complicated grief that never goes away, and keeps resurfacing every time there is a change to our functioning or changed relationships.

If grief counselling was offered as a part of our 'treatment or ongoing support and management' very soon after diagnosis, as it would be for any other terminal illness, I feel reasonably confident a lot fewer people with dementia would be diagnosed with depression and apathy.

One of the reactions of having been diagnosed with dementia for at least the first couple of years was I immediately started beating the mathematical or statistical odds. What I mean by that is that suddenly I was the one that was always wrong…had forgotten the appointment… left the lunch box on the kitchen cupboard…forgotten visitors were coming…lost the shopping list…lost the ****…you get my drift!

Suddenly, it was always my fault, even though initially my memory loss was less of a feature, and was only episodic and very random memory loss. Even now, some family members will say to me after I've said I can't recall something or someone from our family history or stories: 'Don't be silly, of course you remember!'

Quite frankly, sometimes I do, sometimes I do not.

When you are a child, you are taught telling a lie is wrong. In my case, I was also told it was a sin, and if caught lying or swearing, we would have a bar of soap rubbed onto our teeth. It is difficult for me to lie, although often now I just agree with people, or their insistence that I remember things, to stop the arguments. In fact, I have often wondered, is this the beginning of confabulation?

The responses of others vary; some are overprotective, immediately wanting to help you, take over for you, trying to love you more to make up for the diagnosis.

Others have openly suggested or accused me of lying; if you can still speak and function, then you can't have it, or maybe you are lying for notoriety or sympathy. Many others with dementia speak of this, and I know of some who carry letters from the neurologist as proof, or use pictures of their own brain scans within their public presentations, calling them their 'credibility' slides. Some, me included, have had doctors say our diagnosis is wrong, or the scans must be stolen if they have been used in a presentation. This is despite the fact that numerous medical opinions have been requested, and annual follow-up tests are carried out. If we can still speak and function as we do, all of our doctors are wrong, or we are lying. This used to be hugely upsetting, but these days I simply suggest they attend my next neurologist appointment, and offend their own colleagues!

Unfortunately, the lack of in-depth knowledge that many doctors, nurses and care partners actually have of dementia is, for many, still seriously scary. Undergraduate education spends too little time on it too, and for the most part postgraduate education in dementia is still lacking and underwhelming.

It always makes me wonder what it is about dementia that brings such disbelief; if we were diagnosed with cancer and doing well, others would be applauding us for our efforts, whether they be Western medical or holistic or a combination of both, and asking us what we were doing, rather than accusing us of lying.

If we had been cured of cancer or some other fatal disease through a God miracle, even the atheist and agnostic doctors would believe it. As Dr Ross Walker, an eminent cardiologist in Australia, says, even without evidence-based research to prove it, if a patient of his gets well, whether through holistic, God or other interventions, how can he dispute the facts? And yet, when it comes to dementia, that is rarely the response.

The other very hurtful part of living with dementia is that many of our friends simply do not want to engage in our journey, and if we aren't able to fit into their world any more, we are simply left out. I know this also happens a lot to people who lose a partner, and suddenly become 'single'. Some have actively told us they do not wish to learn more about what is happening…or share it with us. They have quietly walked away, perhaps having no idea of how much this hurts. I remain hopeful that is the case…

Many others say, 'but I forget things too' or 'my mother/ father is like that'. Then if you remember something in a conversation, some will say, 'see, you can't possibly have dementia', even though not everyone with dementia has memory loss, and certainly in the early stages, there is rarely a total lack of memory recall.

My youngest son Charles said, 'But Mum, isn't that a funny old person's disease!'

But no-one laughed…

None of us had ever considered younger people are also diagnosed with dementia, not even me, and I had worked in aged care and then, ironically, the first secure dementia unit in Adelaide in 1977.

My mother said in an interview (Collins 2009), when she found out I had been diagnosed with dementia, that she felt an anger she had never felt before, one that eventually subsided, but which left her with a deep, deep sadness.

Some time ago now, my husband Peter said in an email between us: 'I know I am losing you, and I am afraid of what the future holds.'

Many have said nothing. They have quite simply disappeared from our lives. Others hung out with us for a while, but when the going got too tough, they too disappeared. I'm sure this is not through malice or ill will, but is a sign of the ignorance about dementia in the community, and of the stigma still being experienced. But, thankfully, not all.

A group of very special friends have not disappeared, and I also feel lucky to have made a lot of new colleagues and friends in the global dementia community. I love you all.

On many days, I feel almost at the end of wanting to be an advocate and wanting change for people with dementia; some days it just feels too hard and people are too mean. I've felt battered and bruised, and wondered what the point of it is if, after all this time, people with dementia are still not included in the really important conversations about them, and we are still such a long way from being dementia-friendly. Without my special group of friends and colleagues, and my online global community, I would give up. Although my husband or BUB (Back-Up Brain; to be explained in Chapter 23), will say to me, 'Yes, don't get up and go to that meeting; there will be plenty of other people with dementia there to represent you all!' knowing full well there won't be! He can definitely feel like a hot poker stick, prodding me in the backside to keep going.

On top of that, when we go against the perception of dementia and do well with it, there are then those that don't believe we have it, which is hurtful, unkind, and generally downright ignorant. The ugliest part of having dementia is probably the reactions of others, and the two most hurtful reactions are those who stop spending time with us, and those who don't believe us.

We simply have to learn how to ignore them, not always easy, but 100 per cent necessary to get through each day. The offer to take people to my neurologist appointments remains intact, and so far, the people who have either said to my face (the honest ones), said behind my back (the nasty gossips), or implied I am lying (maybe the passive competitive[1] ones) about the diagnosis have never taken me up on it. As always, I'd much rather someone criticised or questioned, openly and honestly, and to my face.

----

1   http://kateswaffer.com/2012/06/26/passive-competitive

At a conference in Sydney in the middle of 2014, I had a Chief Executive of an aged care service provider publicly abuse me and challenge my diagnosis, loudly and aggressively. If that happens by people supposedly in the 'know', it is easier to forgive those in the community who don't know any better. This person should have known better, but was obviously feeling threatened because I had seen the need to criticise – not them personally, but their organisation and the convenors of that particular conference. It is certainly discouraging when a so-called 'peak provider' of dementia and aged care is unable to take criticism, but instead attacks in defence. One can only wonder how we will ever progress towards better understanding and better care, if that is the attitude of the people at the top of a service provider organisation.

At another forum some time ago, some of the care partners of people with dementia suggested to some of us we didn't have dementia, even though they had heard presentations from people with dementia about how this is offensive, and how much this hurts. This can only stem from the fact their own experience has been different, or perhaps they feel trapped in the martyr role, with all the power.

In public places, like retail outlets and cafes, if I get confused or forgetful about what I'm are doing or ordering, then you get what can only be called the 'sour lemon look', from people young enough or smug enough not to realise they too might be diagnosed with dementia one day or some other disAbling disease.

Many subconsciously blame the person with dementia for their changed 'behaviours', rather than the disease.

Many forget it is a terminal illness, and we are struggling to come to terms with our own mortality, and struggling to paddle to get through each moment of every single day.

The symptoms of dementia can sometimes get in the way of compassion and often we are 'blamed' for our 'behaviours'. We are blamed for being obstinate, or difficult, or for refusing to acknowledge we have dementia, or for not accepting help, or for mistrusting those who are trying to help, or…or…or…

There are so many times I read or hear about the care partner blaming the person with dementia, rather than the disease, or their own inability to understand our needs, for 'their' troubles and the 'burden' we have become. In many cases, people with dementia are also blamed for the changed roles of family members as they have to take on the role of family 'carer'.

It takes time for family and friends to see it is not us, but the disease. Perhaps some never do.

The overly protective responses are the easiest to cope with, as at least these people don't accuse you of lying, they don't blame the changes on you, and their reactions are truly coming from a place of love and compassion. It is a normal response when a person you love is troubled or ill to want to help them.

After presenting to a group of registered nurses working in the dementia community care sector on the positive psychosocial and non-pharmacological interventions for dementia that I have embraced, one very concerned nurse sat me down afterwards and 'kindly' informed me: 'You do realise, no matter what you do, it [dementia] will get you in the end!'

I have to say, I did not find that helpful, or kind at all, and although I realise those interventions are not a cure, they have certainly improved my sense of wellbeing and quality of life, and there is emerging research that shows many of these interventions do indeed slow down the progression of the disease. Being told it will get me in the end was mildly traumatic, and definitely a negative response to someone trying to live the best life possible with dementia.

Dementia impacts a lot of things, including how you cope with things like grief and stress. In 2013 I had a few days of trauma following being bullied by three people at a family function. It was almost teenage school-yard gangster style, two in a smiling passive aggressive way, one person openly nasty to me and in front of others.

Thanks (?!) to Larry, otherwise known as Mr Dementia in my house, I am no longer able to hold my own in situations like this, and consequently spent many days afterwards crying into my tissues. I got over it, and as always have learned some life lessons from it, but having dementia makes these things much more difficult at the time and afterwards.

One very special friend visited me the next day and held my heart gently in her hands...no words or questioning, simply sitting with me in love and friendship. This is what people with dementia need more than anything else – people to hold their hearts and hands gently and lovingly, no questioning, no-one saying things like 'but I'm like that' or 'you don't have dementia', and especially no-one blaming or judging you for the symptoms or changes in you caused by the disease, or misunderstandings, or treating you badly knowing you are no longer able to stand up for yourself.

The media often cite research that implies blame towards the person diagnosed with dementia as if it is their fault they have it; for example, if you are diagnosed, you must be overweight, a smoker, be a heavy drinker or drug addict, and the most odious is you must be undereducated. These reactions or labels to dementia are deeply offensive, and they have been supported by research projects, perhaps done in lower socio-economic areas, but the full facts of the research are not highlighted when the media report on it.

I wrote a chapter titled 'You Live Until You Die' (2012d) in a book *Learning Life from Illness Stories*, and want to add a précis of that chapter here as it sets the scene of where I've been and how the medical community, whilst very necessary, are in my humble opinion not the font of all knowledge, medical (or otherwise), and that sometimes their arrogance and absolute belief in science gets in the way of diagnosing and of treating not just illness, but the whole person. This is not to say I don't have great respect for doctors, but I feel they have failed me many times, and self-managing in positive ways has more often trumped as far as combating or reducing symptoms of any illness, and of increasing my wellbeing, not only with dementia.

Learning Life from Illness Stories brings together the stories of 14 people who have lived with serious illness, either their own or that of a loved one. The authors reflect on the wisdom they have found in the stories of others, especially, as a common text, *Illness: the Cry of the Flesh* by Havi Carel (2008). They respond to Carel's key questions: Can I be ill and happy? How can I have a good life while living with illness? The authors share their own experiences of pain, grief and despair, and of love, hope, seeking happiness, writing poetry, practising yoga, praying and protesting. This is a book about courage, about finding strength and sources of joy in hard times. It will inspire anyone seeking meaning in the chaos of their own difficult circumstances.

Within my chapter in *Learning Life from Illness Stories* I wrote, 'There is a thin veil between people with illness being treated with dignity or being treated like morons.' I still believe this to be the case.

Bruce Rumbold, Director, Palliative Care Unit, LaTrobe University, Melbourne, Australia, said in his review of *Learning Life from Illness Stories*: 'A fascinating study of the way one authentic narrative – in this case Havi Carel's – can evoke the stories of others… This book, in important ways, witnesses to the diversity and complexity that overlie the universal human story of encounter with finitude.'

Les Todres, Professor of Health Philosophy, Bournemouth University in the UK, said: 'This book offers something important and rare: a demonstration of the kind of scholarship that practises conversational community, is existentially instructive, and touches our common humanity.'

A friend and colleague Dr Sheila Clark, who has specialised in grief in her medical practice for over 20 years, wrote the following review for the journal *Australian Family Physician*. I felt it important to add it as it highlights how important the impact of being told of a serious illness is to patients and their families, which in my experience, doctors and health care service providers spend far too little time considering.

Have you ever contemplated what it must be like for our patient to leave the surgery after we have given a diagnosis of a life-threatening illness? What will they have to face in the coming weeks and months? How will they deal with the loss of their future, their hopes and their dreams, and the threat of annihilation and death?

This unusual book is a collection of remarkable stories of such experiences, told in prose and poetry by ten writers who each have a life-threatening illness such as MS and dementia, or who are confronted by the illness and death of a close family member.

Each story reveals a unique struggle through grief, darkness and despair, of coming to terms with the diagnosis, and of discovering some deep learning from their experience. As one writer puts it, 'Illness, it seems, is a powerful transitional space where it is possible to connect with our inner selves and develop.' In different ways the stories grapple with the existential questions of life and death through philosophy, spirituality, reason and humour.

This is a book for us as doctors: for us to listen to the cry behind the text and to hear our own inner response; then to allow that response to connect us with our patient more empathically and with more understanding, as we walk alongside them through the journey of their illness.

It is also a book for our patient: because it can help them understand that they are not alone, that there are others out there who have 'been there' and that their own experiences are normal. It can be liberating to discover a community of fellow sufferers, who have found a way to face life and with whom to connect through common experience.

Ultimately, it is a book for all of us when we confront our own mortality.

I found these stories very humbling and moving. The courage of each of the writers wells up throughout the pages: courage not only in facing their new reality, but also in sharing publically their profound learnings about life. This book makes me think again about how I relate to my own patients: one of the authors posed the challenging question, 'Why is it that not until you are dying do service providers show their care for the person rather than the disease?'

(Clark 2013, p.252)

I am really proud to be one of the chapter authors in that book, and really hope this new book of mine about my experience of living with dementia in some small way replicates what we as authors tried to do in that one. If it gives people with dementia insight or inspiration to live a better life, I will feel like I have achieved something truly grand, or if it helps even one person feel not so alone, then I will also have more than succeeded.

Within my chapter in *Learning Life from Illness Stories* I explored my quest for the meaning of life and desire to make the footprint I leave behind gentle and meaningful, as I am confronted by the lessons of illness and dying. My energy levels are still often low and this book is being written more in the style of a creative non-fiction account of my experience of dementia and illness, as I search for what is inside my soul and heart. The grief and loss of chronic illness and dying is profound, but the beauty and lessons I am learning far outweigh the sadness.

Most of this narrative focuses on living with dementia, and I hope to address this in a way that is thoughtful, honest and caring. As I work towards these goals, my soul is preparing for the journey of its life, and my soul mate is often quietly crying on the inside. Havi Carel's book *Illness* (2008) has given me insight, as well as validating some of my own feelings and reactions to illness.

In the *Living with Memory Loss* course my husband and I did at Alzheimer's Australia in Adelaide South Australia, of the five people with dementia attending, two of us 'came out' almost immediately to our family and friends, and both experienced a significant drop in our friendships, and in fact a large proportion of them did not respond at all, and have not been in touch since.

Then there was one chap who refused to believe he had dementia, and often said he had no idea why he was attending this group. On the day he arrived in his pyjamas, he almost admitted perhaps he had a problem, especially when we joked with him by saying at 2pm in the afternoon, and it not being a pyjama party, then perhaps it was inappropriate to come along in his PJs.

It is clear everyone responds to the diagnosis in their own way, and many find this diagnosis particularly difficult to come to terms with, in part because of the stigma and discrimination, and in part because of the shame and humiliation we feel when diagnosed. I am hopeful that through speaking out, and through advocating loudly for changes to things like the language used about people with dementia, which I will discuss in more depth in Chapter 19, this will change and people with dementia will feel less ashamed and stigmatised.

For me, writing stories and poetry has been a reaction to dementia, especially poetry. It allows me to explore my feelings, and to filter those feelings by cutting the words down into shorter poems such as haikus. I think this is not so much a reaction or response to dementia, but an effect of the type of dementia I have, a new creativity that is coming from within.

My dear husband Peter and I use humour, and try to laugh at the 'symptoms' of dementia as they come into our lives. This is our 'reaction to dementia'.

We find our attitude is the one very small thing that can make the biggest difference. If you find you are not happy or at least at peace with yourself and the world, then you need to change something.

CHAPTER 8

The Burden of Disbelief

TALKING

Talking
Takes the edge off sadness

Talking
Lets you share your pain

Talking
Makes you feel less alone

(SWAFFER 2012C, P.42)

It seemed such a long, dark road to sanity. So many times the light at the end of the tunnel was hiding; teasing and tempting me into believing it was over, the branches of darkness so often trying to trap me and finally convince me eternal nothingness would be better than this constant nagging search for meaning. Of course sanity is not really a state; it is just a stupid word, full of stigma and mystery, enticing us into taking sides between the black and white rather than accept the grey, where sanity and insanity fade awkwardly and unforgivably into an illusion. This was my reaction to the first years of my life, faced with living in a remote farming community, and then living with chronic illness, the symptoms of which were not believed for many years.

Illness and dementia have given me the gift of understanding, of insight, of meaning, and the certainty of my own sanity.

The hereditary condition I was born with remained undiagnosed for 46 years. The symptoms began in my pre-teens, but I was always told they were not real; they included headaches, occasional dizziness and fainting, and mild intermittent parasthesia, things that no-one could *see*. At the age of 14, when I fell from a horse and injured my fifth cervical vertebrae with a hairline fracture, then at last some of my symptoms were believed. As my life progressed I continued to have increasing parasthesia in my limbs, pain and severe chronic headaches and 'fainting spells' but I was constantly told I was neurotic, an over-achiever, over-stressed, going through a bad patch, a liar, a hypochondriac…or worse.

Mostly I managed, eventually coping with the technique of denial, and finally by forcing myself to ignore my symptoms, and building up a huge pain tolerance. When eventually doctors could not deny something was wrong, they discovered I was born with a rare brain abnormality known as Arnold Chiari Malformation Type 1. This not only explained my lifelong symptoms, but required moderately urgent neurosurgery. Relief was one thing I felt; anger at the medical profession another. Of interest is I then had significantly more difficulty ignoring the symptoms whilst waiting for the surgery; it was as if a floodgate was opened by the acknowledgement of a *real* medical condition.

The fact that doctors have not been willing to believe me has been a persistent pattern in my life. When I fell pregnant after numerous failed pregnancies, the radiologist conducting my earliest scan of this fourth and unexpected pregnancy mentioned I had an anterior placenta praevia, but then forgot to put it in the report. Many times, I mentioned this to my obstetrician, who said I must have 'baby brain' and refused to believe me. Then, at about 32 weeks gestation when I started to haemorrhage and it became an emergency, it was *discovered* I had an anterior placenta praevia! Again, I was not the one who was surprised.

Following the neurosurgery, it was once again a case of doctors not believing in, or devaluing the difficulty of some new symptoms, until finally I was diagnosed with severe urge incontinence; I simply do not get the message from my brain to urinate or defecate. Managing and 'surviving' incontinence is done by following a strict and timed toileting schedule, and wearing continence pads. I had been struggling with this problem for almost two years before it was taken seriously. My incontinence appears to be one of the side effects of the neurosurgery although I have never been given a definitive answer on this, and it was unfortunately also initially treated very glibly. Living with incontinence is not fun, and the wearing of pads humiliating and embarrassing. Not only does it negatively impact one's life in general, it also plays havoc with one's sex life and intimacy and is extremely challenging to live with. Sadly, continence pad companies are selling us short, especially women, telling us 'LBL' (light bladder leakage) is normal even in our twenties and thirties, as a way to sell product, when in fact for most incontinence a strict regime of pelvic floor exercises would prevent it altogether. Oops...another mini rant! Sorry! When my problem was eventually taken seriously, and the diagnosis was confirmed, once again I was not the one who was surprised.

Being diagnosed with dementia is a traumatic event, and in many ways can be the ultimate roller-coaster event of one's life. I know of many who have had the type of their dementia changed, making it even more confusing, for example, initially diagnosed with Alzheimer's disease, then the diagnosis is changed to another 'type' of dementia. Some have eventually been told they don't have dementia, but some other cause for their cognitive impairment and memory loss. Being misdiagnosed, or not diagnosed at all when there really is something wrong, is difficult to deal with emotionally.

One of the greatest challenges of being misdiagnosed, apart from the fact if it was with a terminal illness or very serious chronic condition, and you have grieved for what is happening and ahead of you, is that just as you are coming to terms with the diagnosis and your changed future, and have told your family and friends, it is difficult then to have to tell them your doctor was wrong.

If it happens more than once, then after a while it probably seems to them like you are 'crying wolf'. They may think you are a hypochondriac, or have something more serious like Münchausen syndrome, which is a psychiatric factitious disorder wherein those affected feign or invent disease, illness, or psychological trauma to draw attention, sympathy or reassurance to oneself. I know people with this disorder, and have also seen how the internet and 'Dr Google' almost encourages it. I also know I do not have it.

Part of writing about the numerous times I have either been misdiagnosed or not believed is perhaps my way of proving it to others. I've been misdiagnosed or not believed and not been believed with the very real symptoms of other serious conditions. Frustration is one word that comes to mind, but there are others sounding far more like expletives that popped into my head at the time, definitely not printable here.

The odd thing about being diagnosed with dementia is there is disbelief of the diagnosis at all, if you are not at the end stage of the disease process. The myth that everyone with dementia has profound memory loss and can't fend for themselves is also widespread.

The belief that the symptoms cannot be slowed down by exercise or other healthy interventions, or working hard on non-pharmacological and positive psychosocial interventions to delay the progression of dementia, is wrong. Research is now proving otherwise, and brain health is recommended as pre- and post-vention for dementia, in the same way as healthy lifestyle is recommended for heart disease. Simply because many of us around with world with dementia believed this before there was evidence to prove it does not mean we were or are wrong, or that we are lying about the diagnosis of dementia. It's just that research has not caught up with us!

Arrogance

The superiority and arrogance of many in the health sector continues to astound. Too many twenty-first century doctors and nurses are there for the diseases and not for their patients. They are modern men and women who have taken the science of health too far, and are more interested in being able to diagnose and treat with pharmacology or surgery, rather than being interested in the overall welfare of and outcomes for their patients. Then, if there are no pharmacological or surgical treatment options available, more often than not they are no longer interested in you.

I have been talked down to, or not talked to at all if my husband is there.

My intellect and background was not initially taken into account, my level of intelligence not considered in the initial neuropsychology testing done for dementia. There has been a gross underestimation of the level of my cognitive impairment, and the disAbilities caused by them, because I am still externally reasonably functional. When one of my specialists had diagnosed motor neurone disease, a disease where it was expected I would die a very speedy and untimely death, my general practitioners and all other health providers became openly caring. A palliative health care team moved in, and were truly interested in me as a person, and how they could support me and my family, rather than just making notes about the disease. They sought not to confirm pain or other symptoms through tests, but to believe respectfully and treat accordingly.

I am still searching for the answer to this question: why is it not until you are dying that most doctors and health care providers show their care for the whole person, not just the disease? I doubt I will ever find the answer…

Like Havi Carel, I found phenomenology helpful 'as it privileges the first-person experience, thus challenging the medical world's objective, third-person account of disease' (2008, p.8). She also talks of cynicism (p.49); I am reasonably cynical, although work on trying not to become too cynical as I believe that would negatively impact me, and it is not necessarily helpful in bringing about change. Instead I have chosen to speak out as an activist and advocate for those living with chronic illness like dementia and for those in aged care, sitting inside what I often call *'the human cattle yards for aged care and dementia'*. Places where people I have loved once had to live, and where many others have also told me it feels like being locked in a prison or a concentration camp.

We all live until we die; some of us simply prefer to do the living part as positively as humanly possible.

This is in spite of the fact that living with dementia is like watching on as my world disappears, slipping away from me. I once felt losing my legs and arms or my eyes, or even contracting AIDS, would be better than this disease, one I once thought of as hideous and a death sentence. After diagnosis, the tears ran down my cheeks for many weeks, the tang of salt a permanent fixture on my tastebuds. I thought: *If only someone would tell me it is just depression or some bizarre mental illness...anything other than dementia.* It was confirmed I had not had a stroke, there were no signs of post-operative bleeding from the brain surgery and no signs of a brain tumour; *good news* they told me, as if having dementia was okay.

In fact, during the last few years, I have discovered living with dementia is okay, although not in the way they meant at that time!

The changes brought on by dementia are relentless, yet most people do not see them as disAbilities but rather only see the external symptoms; and if they can't see external symptoms, then they think you don't have dementia. As mentioned earlier, many also think it is a mental illness, which it is not.

The word dementia is taken from Latin, originally meaning 'madness'; no wonder we struggle against the myths! And so, we are regularly defined by the symptoms of our disease: forgetful, confused, aggressive, odd behaviour, absconders or refusing to communicate, rather than the people we still are…mothers, fathers, lovers, daughters, wives or husbands, employees or employers, grandmothers, aunties.

It is a tragedy that so many just see our deficits.

CHAPTER 9

Being Diagnosed with Younger Onset Dementia

What matters in life is not what happens to you but what you remember and how you remember it.

(GABRIEL GARCÍA MÁRQUEZ)

What is younger onset dementia (YOD)?

I've written this chapter specifically about younger onset dementia, because that is what I have. It is not a detailed clinical description of it, but about my lived experience.

Younger onset dementia is simply the diagnosis of a person under the age of 65 with a dementia, sometimes also referred to as early onset dementia. It varies, but the impact of dementia on a person under 65 is significantly different to the impact on someone over the age of 65.

A diagnosis of dementia at any age, above or below 65, affects thinking, behaviour and the ability to perform everyday tasks. Brain function is affected enough to interfere with the person's normal social or working life. It is the gradual deterioration of functioning, such as thinking, concentration, memory, and judgement, which affects a person's ability to perform normal daily activities.

There are estimated to be more than 25,800 Australians currently living with younger onset dementia but there are very few age-appropriate services to cater for our specific needs. Through targeted promotion and advocacy, my aim is to raise the profile of the illness and the impact it has on those of us of any age diagnosed with it.

The impact of a diagnosis of YOD

Although the symptoms of dementia are similar whatever a person's age, younger people with dementia experience many issues different to someone over the age of 65. The following is a list of the issues I have seen, although it is not exhaustively based on any individual's experience:

- Prescribed Disengagement® (see Chapter 16 for an explanation of this term).

- Usually still in paid employment, and there is no support to remain employed.

- Once we have to give up paid employment, usually recommended straight away, our family income often halves as we become a single or no income family.

- May have dependent children still living at home, and in some cases very young children.

- Child care may be required because of the person with dementia not being able to care for their own children, and their partner having to work.

- Have significant financial commitments.

- Physically fit and may behave in ways that others find challenging.

- More aware of their disease in the early stages.

- Find it hard to accept and cope with losing skills at such a young age.

- Find it difficult to access information, as support and services are targeted to people over 65.

- Have a partner who is still in full-time employment.

- Health costs can more than double.

- Travel costs, to accommodate health care appointments and other services required, increase.

- Often have the rarer types of dementia (such as frontotemporal or Lewy body).

- Our symptoms are not seen as disAbilities, but as deficits.

- Reduced self-worth as our valued roles are diminished or negated.

- Increased risk of depression, low self-esteem, anxiety.

- There are very few or no age-appropriate services. Therefore many of the Aged Accreditation Standards are currently being breached in the (Australian) residential setting.

- We may no longer be able to drive; this impacts us in a number of ways, including not being able to pick up our own children from school, take them or ourselves to medical or other appointments; they may not be able to take elderly parents to appointments or on outings, and so on, and their partner (if they have one) becomes less able to work as they are required to assist with more.

- Unequal social status.

- The impact of the diagnosis of dementia is treated differently to other terminal illnesses, and no support services are set up as they would be for other terminal illnesses.

- The loss and grief caused by a diagnosis of dementia is often under-recognised and under-treated, and complicated.

- Significant fear of a loss of identity, the loss of privacy, of not knowing your children or grandchildren.

- Means-tested care partner allowance is not only unreasonable, it is not cost effective.

- The negative impact, and the physical and emotional burden on their children, spouse and older parents, as caregivers, becomes significant.

- Lack of support for meaningful engagement and pre-diagnosis activities.

Anthea Innes, in her book *Dementia Studies* (2009), claims further studies need to look at the micro level of experiences of dementia patients themselves, and must move beyond current research and policies, to establish services and support for real wellbeing, rather than to support current polices and services provided in the care settings.

Perhaps the other most significant missing link for people with younger onset dementia is age-specific support and services.

Aged care standards and YOD

In Australia, the Aged Care Assessment Team (ACAT) age discriminates against people with younger onset dementia and I think it could be more helpful if the term was changed to Disability Care Assessment Team. It is very difficult for someone with younger onset dementia to access services in the aged care sector because technically services start at 65; nor is it easy to find residential care in the disAbility sector as this cuts out at the age of 50. Policy is changing in Australia, and currently it seems as though it is going to become more difficult to access services if you are under the age of 65.

If a residential *aged* care facility accepts me, they are probably in breach of at least ten Australian Aged Care Accreditation standards. I am a 57-year-old woman, and there is one 12-bed, age-appropriate residential facility interstate for respite or residential care specific to someone my age, and although not listed here, thankfully more are emerging.

There are accreditation standards to providing care, and currently if I enter an aged care facility that does not have an age-specific – and appropriate to my age – unit or wing, I believe the nursing home will be breaking no less than ten of the Australian Aged Care Accreditation Standards, because of my age. For example, we would not place children in the geriatric or adult ward in a hospital, but into a specialised paediatric ward. This breach of a duty of care towards people with younger onset dementia appears to have been completely overlooked by the government, aged care facilities and, importantly, the Accreditation Board.

In a submission I made to a Federal Government Inquiry (Swaffer 2011b), I reported that there are a number of standards a residential aged care facility would contravene when residents under 65 years of age are residing permanently or in respite, as follows.

From the Australian Accreditation Standards:[1]

Standard 2: Health and Personal Care

2.12 Lack of appropriate continence management, and instead the necessity by neglect of the use of continence aids

2.15 Oral and dental care cannot be provided if the resident does not have suitable mobility to travel to a dentist as there is no dental service available on site

Standard 3: Resident Lifestyle

3.4 Emotional support requirements differ to the aged person

3.5 Independence changes – not easy to maintain friendships and participate in life of the facility due to significant age differences

3.6 Dignity may be impaired due to relationships are only available with residents with significant age differences

3.7 Leisure activities set up for the elderly, not people under 65

3.8 Very different lifestyle, age related cultural backgrounds and values

3.9 Impaired choice and decision making as no matter how much control they may be able to exercise, the choices available are specific to the elderly

Standard 4: Physical Environment and Safe Systems

4.4 Living environment set up and aesthetically suitable for older residents

4.8 Catering provision is targeted to the taste requirements of a different generation, and to residents who may be far more impaired physically.

---

1   www.aacqa.gov.au/for-providers/accreditation-standards

Residential care facilities talk about, but do not yet deliver, person-centred care as the norm, and many people there feel as if they have been locked in prison. Reassurance that they are not in prison, and that they have been moved for their own safety and care, does not serve to stop them feeling like they are in prison. The activities, the day room, the dining rooms, are full of people who all seem to be suffering from what Martin Luther King called *a sense of nobodiness* as they are herded together to allow facilities to work more efficiently, and to ensure the perceived provision of better care (King 1963). Imagine being 30 and living there, although my father-in-law and other friends and family felt equally wronged about having to live in aged care for their final days.

It is very encouraging to see this is changing, and the aged care sector in general is making a huge effort to embrace change, and to provide better care, including age-appropriate care.

Dementia brings with it a very complicated grief, as discussed in more detail in Chapter 12. Our children, partners and parents are impacted differently, and have an increased challenge of having to become our supporters or BUBs (Back-Up Brains; see Chapter 23), and our partner has an increased financial load due to our lost employment, and often theirs. We are definitely told to give up work too early. If I was given assistance and support, known legally as Reasonable Adjustments, in the same way as if I had sustained an injury following a car accident, I would have been offered rehabilitation and given every chance to stay at work for as long as possible. Our income is reduced because the family income usually halves in a family with a person with younger onset dementia, as both adults are often working, or if living alone, then many will become dependent on the government or others for financial support.

Our health costs increase as do our travel costs when we lose our driver's licence.

Self-esteem and self-confidence is battered, and yes, as already mentioned, many friendships disappear.

Many people with dementia are actively involved, as members or consultants (unpaid), on international, national and local committees. For example, I worked with Resthaven and Uniting Communities for almost 18 months helping them review and change their aged and dementia care; I am currently working with many other organisations doing the same. I have been a keynote speaker all over the world, and all over Australia. I currently sit on various Alzheimer's Australia and other international, national and state committees. I'm writing this book about my experience of dementia and currently have a second and third volume of poetry about to be published. I completed a Master's of Science in Dementia Care in 2014. Of course I am still capable of paid work, although I would and do require a lot of disAbility support. When I was working in a paid consulting role with appropriate disAbility support, I was able to function well still. It was economically and emotionally very destructive to have been told to give up paid employment upon diagnosis and the economic cost to governments and society in general has never been considered formally.

Younger onset vs older onset dementia

Often I am discussing with others about the impact of younger onset dementia being different to that of older onset dementia, and am regularly told, 'What a load of bollocks, older people have as many things to lose as you do.' I disagree, and I do think, in some ways, it is more emotionally challenging and I feel sure many of the losses are very different. I've even been called ageist because of it, and also because I feel it is unreasonable that someone my age (with any condition or illness where residential care is required), should be placed in *aged* care. Perhaps in the same way as dying from cancer aged 24 or 48 as opposed to dying from cancer aged 75 is. We do have more life and living to lose, and therefore more lost dreams. The idea of not seeing our children reach 21, or marry, or not meeting our grandchildren, is distressing, and although older people lose their dreams too, they have experienced so many more of the dreams and experiences people with younger onset dementia are often very expectantly anticipating. Ask my sons... I have been nagging them to have children since they turned 18, as I can hardly wait to be a grandmother!

Imagine being diagnosed with dementia in your twenties or thirties. I think it would be worse not only for the person diagnosed, but also for their children and parents – far worse than it was for me aged 49. This is also true for any terminal illness or serious chronic condition. Suffice to say, it is not a competition of how horrible it can be, merely recognition it is different.

For older people, I imagine losing a partner you might have been married to for over 60 years is worse, and definitely different, than when you are younger. The longer I am with my husband, I know, the more we 'know' each other, without having to say anything, and, I suspect, the more I would miss him. I lost someone I loved at the age of 27, but still had a long life ahead of me to heal, and to regroup and find love again – even though it did not feel like that at the time. I have some older friends who felt like they had been 'forced to separate' when the husband went into aged care, and they mourned for their marriage and the loss of living together as a couple.

The losses and issues people with dementia of any age face vary significantly, and are always unique to every individual, but I felt it worthwhile highlighting some of the differences someone diagnosed with dementia under the age of 65 might experience.

Even though I had worked as a nurse in a dementia unit in 1977, I had no idea younger people could be diagnosed with dementia. Mostly, the impact of my own diagnosis was one of great shock.

CHAPTER 10

Children of People with Younger Onset Dementia

In 2014 I attended a workshop in Sydney with my youngest son about the impact of younger onset dementia (YOD) on our children. The day was facilitated by Karen Hutchinson, a Research Master's Student based at the Cognitive Decline Partnership Centre, University of Sydney. I had not heard my son speak openly about having a mother diagnosed with dementia, and wept throughout most of the day and for many days following the event. Many other young people spoke courageously and candidly about the impact having a parent with dementia had on them, at the time and since. There were stories of drug and alcohol abuse, mental illness, and homelessness; some talked of a total disengagement from the world they had known to one of invisibility and fear; escape was often seen by young people as the only choice. The overwhelming reaction following this day was that if I thought services were very sparse for me, I should have been one of them!

There was some interesting data presented by Karen that came out of this workshop. At the time, it was estimated that in Australia there were 24,400 people living with YOD which is 6–9 per cent of all dementia cases in Australia. In comparison the Australian data estimated 23,300 people living with multiple sclerosis, a very similar population size but no comparison as to level of public awareness. A Norwegian study published in 2014 estimated that a third of people with YOD had a family member under 18 years and most pertinent to this chapter there was *no data on the number of young people impacted by dementia in any study* (Barca *et al.* 2014). Many of the young people in Karen's study reported feeling alone, thinking no-one else had a family similar to them, and had no idea where to get help from.

The following is part of a media release titled 'Diagnosis of younger onset dementia has life changing impact on families', published during Dementia Awareness Month 2014:

> A diagnosis of younger onset dementia is not only challenging for the person who receives the diagnosis but has an enormous impact on the entire family. Currently there are no official figures as to how many young people in families are impacted in Australia.
>
> Isolation and guilt are the overwhelming feelings, according to children of a parent with younger onset dementia at the recent Supporting Young People Having a Parent with Younger Onset Dementia Workshop.
>
> Karen Hutchinson, workshop organiser and author of the recent paper 'The emotional well-being of young people having a parent with younger onset dementia', published in *Dementia,* told workshop attendees, that *children of a parent living with younger onset dementia are often the invisible care partners and are not recognised by health care providers.*
>
> 'Our study identified four common experiences of young people living with a parent with younger onset dementia,' said Karen Hutchinson. 'These included the emotional toll

of caring, keeping the family together, grief and loss and psychological distress.'

Presenters told the workshop of feelings of disengagement, anger and despair when a parent was diagnosed with YOD.

'There was a big change in the way people treated me when they found out my mother had dementia. Nobody was giving me guidance or monitoring my behaviour,' explained one young person who had a parent diagnosed with younger onset dementia.

'Support from extended family disappears and friends disappear due to the stigma associated with dementia. People don't know how to deal with someone with dementia and distance themselves.'

'We need to look at how we better engage with young people of parents with younger onset dementia to inform them of the numerous channels of support out there. It was good to hear about the services available, and I hope that there will be growth of this support in the future.'

Mark Gaukroger, who at the time was the Director of Dementia policy at the Department of Health and Ageing, said: 'The most important thing is the sustainability of the care partners and the access to all the support services. We have gained a much greater understanding that dementia is not solely a health issue but has huge social implications.'

I wrote this about the impact of younger onset dementia on my children in 2012:

It was a tough day when I had to tell my school age children I had dementia, something we all thought was an 'old person's' disease. They were probably as confused as I was, but because I had been through a lot of other health issues, for them it was more of a roller-coaster, just another thing to go wrong in our family. As I have progressed, albeit slowly, they have had to learn to cope in the best way they can. It is difficult for them to have a mother who forgets things or can't work things out sometimes. For years, they even think we know everything!! When they are young, children rely on us for everything, help with homework, transport to and from things, shopping, being taken to the doctor and sporting events, and so on. Now that this is not possible, and whilst it is awful, I have no choice but to find other ways to support them. As a mother, I feel guilt and sadness that I am not there for them in the way I used to be. I am only glad they were almost finished their schooling and not babies or in primary school, as some children of parents with YOD are, as that would be so much worse.

But, it seems, this was still too much about me! Having a mother with dementia, and then an elderly grandparent in residential high care, was difficult for my children. When their grandad was at home, they willingly visited him, and even when he went into residential low-care, they were okay about visiting. However, once he went into high care, they were too confronted to visit, as the thought of their mother being in an *aged* care facility was too much for them to cope with. This is one of the more subtle challenges for children of having a parent with younger onset dementia. And then when he died, they both spoke of the guilt of not having been to see grandad. It was poignant and desperately sad.

The books and resources for children are almost exclusively based around a grandparent having dementia, rather than a mother or father with YOD, and therefore it is time we talked about it. If anyone can refer me to a book for children of any age who have a parent with dementia, please do let me know; I'm not sure I'm emotionally capable of writing a book exclusively for children of parents with dementia!

At the time I was diagnosed it was confusing for us all, and perhaps especially so for my children, and I realise now I probably neglected to give them the support they needed, as I was so traumatised by the diagnosis myself. We were all worried about upsetting each other, and became overprotective by trying to hide how we felt. I spent a lot of time walking and running, and, during this time, crying. I could barely stop crying, and this was my escape. Sadly, I realise now it took me away from helping the boys. At the time, there was also very little support for any of us, but less for them than for my husband and me.

When I was first diagnosed, my youngest son said, 'But mum, *I thought dementia was a funny old person's disease?*' He said it casually, and with humour, and we all took it in that way, but the reality for my children is they have a mother who is very slowly deteriorating in front of their eyes. And it is not funny. I'm quite sure it was difficult for both of my teenage sons, who at the time still lived at home, to watch me progress from a highly capable woman to someone who is sometimes 'too scared to leave the house'. Aged 50, I also lost my driver's licence, which meant I could not pick them up from school or sport, or drive them to the doctor or shops, all simple things almost every other parent and child take for granted.

A couple of years ago, my husband was unable to attend the funeral of a friend who died from younger onset dementia, and so one son came with me, partly to take me because I can no longer drive, and partly to support me. Part way through the service, he was crying as much as I was even though he had never met them, and we both hugged and held onto each other tightly. It wasn't until afterwards when we discussed our feelings that I found out why he was so upset. He had felt it was like attending my funeral. I too felt it was a more than a glimpse of what is ahead, and it affected us both deeply. Of course we cannot live in fear every day, but it was and is occasionally very confronting, and makes us all very aware of what is ahead.

My other son held me tightly after the funeral of another friend with younger onset vascular dementia, with the same sense of fear. Like all young people, they get on with their lives, but lurking in their subconscious most of the time is the fear I might one day be in an aged care facility, and will probably die much sooner than we all would want. At times it is desperately sad for everyone; whether it is your grandma, or mother, or friend, if they don't remember you or you are confused even some of the time, it really hurts and can be sad. We tend to live as if every day is our last together, just in case it is, and we are trying to make sure we spend more time together. We always hug and tell each other we love each other, every time we connect.

Whilst neither of my children are technically 'care partners' for me, they do have to be with me sometimes, as well as provide transport. Their lives don't completely revolve around this, but there is probably a sense of 'being on call', in case my husband is not able to help when needed.

It is most likely difficult for them to express their feelings or fears with their own friends, as almost none have a parent with dementia. Many do have grandparents with dementia, so at least there is a common thread of experience, but it is not an easy topic to discuss for anyone, and young people have to date mostly been left out of the conversations. Until very recently, the active support for the children of people with younger onset dementia has almost been ignored. I imagine the idea of talking about the abilities that have 'gone into hiding', and are slowly getting worse, feels like a betrayal of their mother. Accepting the repetition of conversations, and my increasing forgetfulness is also hard for them, and as they don't live with us any more, it is easy for them to forget about dementia, and so they potentially can become more easily frustrated when with me.

Eventually, it may feel like having a parent who is absent, and they may then also have to take on some of the roles and chores of a parent. I read about the effects of this on adult children, who care for their elderly parents, and know many feel like their elderly parent has become the child, and they have become the parent. They write about the intense sense of loss they feel at not having a mother or father capable of fulfilling the roles they had for their whole life, the sadness and grief of not having a parent 'there for them' or to ask for advice from, and the challenges of having to become their 'care partner'. Imagine that, but your mum is 35 or 49.

I have not written a lot about the impact me having a dementia has had on my wonderful husband, Peter, but do know that he struggles with it, and, like me, prefers to stay in the denial bubble as much as is humanly possible. That is also why he doesn't write about his experience. I have heard him say, 'It is just too sad to think about, let alone write about.'

Once, after finding him sitting on the foot of our stairs, looking forlorn and with his head in his hands, when I asked him what was wrong he said, 'I know I am losing you, and I am afraid of what the future holds.'

I wrote a tribute to him on my blog recently, which I would like to share with you here.

A tribute to my BUB

Many people over the last few weeks in the UK have gone up to my husband and said things like; we know you as BUB...do you have a real name?! Peter, also my Back-Up Brain, is my husband and one of my heroes, and I do have him up on a pedestal for the way he manages physically and emotionally to support me living with dementia, in such pro-active and empowering ways. He has said he feels he doesn't deserve the accolades from me or others, but other people with dementia, and family care partners or supporters of people with dementia, often ask us how we maintain our relationship so well and with such affection and how we have managed to negotiate the often very difficult and confronting minefield of changes in our relationship and our lives due to dementia.

How does he manage to not take away all my power and control, and how does he sit back and watch me struggle and not take over or further disable me?

The first couple of years were tough, and we did not have it working well as we had both accepted and assumed the roles that Prescribed Disengagement® ensures most people take on. Perhaps being diagnosed in the earlier stages of dementia and having a lot of insight has helped, or maybe my fiercely independent personality and desire to do things for myself for as long as possible, but it was not an easy road to navigate. He did, often, try to take over for me, and initially I not only let him, I thought he needed to, long before it was really necessary.

In the early days following the diagnosis, I allowed myself to be disabled, and as per the service providers' advice and education, focused on my deficits and the fear of the supposed road to nowhere ahead of us.

Being at the University of SA was most likely the breakthrough that allowed us to see things differently and respond accordingly; they advised me to not only see the symptoms as disAbilities to be managed, but to work hard to accommodate the symptoms of dementia, and see them as disAbilities, even as assets, not as deficits.

Being a pro-active type of person, one who has almost always been able to find solutions in the toughest of situations, has been useful. Resilience, discipline and motivation have been imperative. But my BUB has made all the difference, and I barely have the words to say how much he means to me, and to thank him.

Amongst many other personality traits, I am naturally extremely independent, often to the point of being too proud to ask for help in some really tough situations. I have always rejected 'needing' anyone, even my husband, as I always felt I wanted to live my life as independently and with as many as resources as possible, and that to be needy was unhealthy and unhelpful. Over the last three to four years, this has had to change. In particular this last year or so, I now really need Pete's support and active help.

Due to some physical disAbilities, some completely unrelated to dementia, I can no longer lift or carry many things. I cannot drive, so, for example, during a driving holiday around the UK or anywhere else, this means Pete always has to drive. My list of deficits is growing, and Pete needs to manage the money, as I can't work out the different currencies, and can no longer add or subtract, not even with a calculator.

Even with our connected electronic calendars, I can no longer work out how to add a diary event, and have had to go back to a paper diary, which I often can't find or have forgotten to write appointments in! I often cannot work out how to set the GPS, or read maps or instructions. I cannot work out how to use new TV controls, and I easily get lost, even in familiar places at home. This does seem, oddly for me, to be focusing on my deficits, but I wanted to highlight just how much help my dear husband has to provide – that I actually need.

My frustration levels are higher than they used to be with many of these things, and having meltdowns is not uncommon. He patiently and quietly puts up with them, rides them out, alongside me, without getting too impatient or angry too often, and at the end of it, insists he still loves me. Now that is one pretty fantastic BUB!

He has never said to me, or to others as far as I know, that he 'hates being my care partner', nor has he ever said he 'didn't sign up for this' when he married me, two lines we have often heard from other family care partners. I feel very lucky!

I love you Peter Watt, and hope you can accept this very deserved public accolade.

CHAPTER 11

Early vs Delayed Diagnosis

What's the rush
Life as I know it
Will always be there
I'll always be able to
Make my own decisions
And brush my own hair
I'll always be able to
And sail through the waves
Remembering my loved ones...
Won't I?

(KATE SWAFFER 2015)

It can take many people years to get a diagnosis of dementia, in fact, many years sometimes for your doctor to take you seriously, and not put your symptoms down to things like depression, menopause, middle age, stress, anxiety or perhaps even more likely possibilities such as post-traumatic stress disorder. Many other conditions also have memory loss or cognitive impairment, many only temporary, some with ongoing cognitive deficits or symptoms. For younger people it can take at least three years to get a confirmed diagnosis, and some have even told me it took them that long just to get a referral to a specialist. Unfortunately, the medical and nursing profession is not as well educated in dementia as they are in most other diseases, and this is an issue that universities and the health sector need to address.

Early or timely diagnosis

The primary purpose and value of early diagnosis of dementia is timely access to information, advice, and support and access to a pathway of effective treatment and care from the time of diagnosis to end-of-life care, and to enable interventions that may only work or be suitable in the earlier stages (Alzheimer's Disease International 2011).

Early diagnosis for people with the symptoms of dementia is essential as they may still have the ability to think logically, even though their powers of reasoning may have started to be impaired. They will more easily be able to discuss the implications of the illness and how it will affect them and their families now and in the future, and it is the time when decisions regarding future care needs and financial and legal issues must be considered, while the person with dementia still has legal capacity.

Giving the diagnosis at this early stage is not that different to the diagnosis of any other chronic and terminal illnesses, in terms of the discussion process. Obviously it is important to remember the person with dementia may already be experiencing memory difficulty, and therefore time must be taken to give the information in ways it can be retained, including repetition, printed information, and having other family members present. Engaging the person with dementia is easier at an early stage because they are more likely to be less impaired with memory and cognition.

People with dementia do have a moral and ethical right to be told of the diagnosis; doctors do not have the right to withhold it, even if a family member asks them to. Ethically, they would not withhold a diagnosis of cancer or any other terminal illness, so it is absolutely unacceptable some believe they have the right to withhold the diagnosis of dementia.

Early diagnosis can empower the person with dementia to improve their own quality of life and may assist them to remain independent for as long as possible. It offers more opportunity for increased and continued social engagement and community participation, and for things like improving lifestyle, rehabilitation and new learning – the three things found to be extremely helpful in risk reduction of dementia.

It allows us to plan for our futures, including organising financial and legal affairs and preparing for longer-term or more intensive care requirements. Early diagnosis helps the person with dementia to be in a position to become active with advocacy and education of and about their condition within their own community. Early diagnosis also allows the best outcomes for activities such as brain training, relearning and retention training (Bier *et al.* 2009; Heredia *et al.* 2009). It also seems clear that the impact of developing a shared social identity among a group of people with early-stage dementia is important in the wellbeing and happiness of these patients (Bright *et al.* 2008).

Early diagnosis and therefore earlier intervention, especially of a person with a younger onset dementia, may also allow the person to stay in paid employment for longer, reducing the cost impact to families, and ultimately governments. It is also vital to delaying institutionalisation, and to the shared welfare of the person with dementia and their loved ones.

Delayed diagnosis

A delayed diagnosis of dementia can reduce choices and shared opportunities with loved ones for many people, and can have a number of significant and negative outcomes:

- Rate of the disease may progress more quickly because of the reduced ability to participate in healthy lifestyle, non-pharmacological and positive psychosocial interventions.

- The person with dementia may no longer have legal capacity to make decisions in their own interests.

- Ability and opportunity to remain in paid employment, with Reasonable Adjustments, may be missed.

- Decreased willingness or ability to participate in social or other activities.

- Reduced ability to accept they have dementia and come to terms with it.

- Impaired ability to go through a healthy grieving process.

- Impaired ability to share end-of-life decisions with their family.

- Impaired ability to make financial decisions.

- Appointing people to make decisions in their best interest may be impaired.

- There may be a conflict of interest between the person with dementia and the person who will end up having to take over their affairs.

- Accepting decisions, such as the loss of their driving licence, is more difficult.

- If medication is available for the type of dementia they are diagnosed with, they might have missed out on the opportunity of the improved quality of life this may give them, albeit only short term.

- Drugs trials may no longer be available to them because of the stage they have entered.

- Family members will lose the opportunity to fully share in the diagnosis, and grieve with their loved one.

- Person with dementia more at risk of physical injury.

- Person with dementia more at risk of getting lost as safety systems not in place.

- Driving may become very dangerous, therefore impact to own and others' safety.

- Insurance policies may be null and void if diagnosis is discovered to have been delayed, and an accident takes place.

- Personal growth that could have been achieved through self-awareness of the disease impaired by late diagnosis.

- Ability to self-advocate, and for socialisation and community involvement impaired.

- Increased isolation.

- Increased loneliness.

- Increased problems with general health.

- Increased visit to the GP because of the 'masking' of dementia symptoms, with obvious cost implications to governments.

- Increased levels of depression, anxiety, anger, and behaviour management requirements.

- Increased costs of care.

(Alzheimer's Disease International 2011, p.8)

Significantly, an early diagnosis of dementia could well reduce stigma and increase awareness about dementia, simply because the community would see more people living beyond dementia in their communities, rather than only seeing people at later stages of the dementia with high levels of impairment.

In my own experience, I sometimes wish I had not been diagnosed early as the level of disbelief in the community of having dementia is often a real burden, and I have wondered, like Richard Taylor, if the devastation and fear caused by things like the stigma might have been prevented with a delayed diagnosis. I used to agree with him, but these days I do feel the best chance of coming to grips with the 'psychological tornado of fears driven by irrational beliefs' he has written about is to be diagnosed earlier into the disease.

But then, I would be cranky if my doctor didn't tell me about having heart disease, diabetes, or cancer, so not wanting to know about a diagnosis of dementia, to me, just doesn't make sense. Knowledge is power, indeed – even a diagnosis of dementia.

CHAPTER 12

Dementia, Grief and Loss: It's Very Complicated

LOSS

Tragedy so great
Illuminating you with sadness
Seems impossible to recover
Lack of lustre lasting forever
Acceptance and healing
A lifetime away
To hear a song or smell a scent
That throws you right back
Into the pit of grief
One step forward
Many steps backwards
From the intensity of sorrow
Meaninglessness, emptiness
Impaired judgments
Damaged relationships
Memories stained with pain
Walls crumbling inside your heart
This journey of grief goes on

(KATE SWAFFER 2014)

Let me begin this chapter with the description of a word I only recently came across, but which I feel sets the scene for this chapter.

'Hiraeth' is a longing for one's homeland; but it's not mere homesickness. It's an expression of the bond one feels with one's home country when one is away from it.

The meaning of the word has been playing with my heart-strings ever since, especially how it relates to dementia, but also around the loss of family and friends after diagnosis, or for that matter a loss or disconnection from family for any reason.

Initially it brought me to tears, as apart from a couple of cousins and two elderly aunts whom I love dearly and speak to reasonably often (although I always tend to feel guilty, as it is never often enough!), my husband and two sons are the only family who actively support me, or are connected to me in any meaningful way. The reality is that some of my immediate family no longer even speak to me at all, and have removed themselves and their children from our lives. It definitely feels like the meaning of the word hiraeth also applies to those losses.

'Their loss, not mine' (or ours) is easy to say, but the impact is much tougher to live with. It is not just on me, but also on my sons who have basically lost close connections with grandparents, cousins, aunts and uncles in the process. I think this is cruel to them in particular, and unacceptable, but understand there are some things I cannot change, no matter how hard I once tried. I have simply had to adjust and heal, which is a constant journey and process needed to deal with the hurt, and ultimately have had to move on with my life without them.

But beyond my immediate family pain and the feelings of hiraeth there, my experience of living with dementia also feels like an experience of hiraeth. Indeed, it does feel like homesickness or a longing for whom and what I once was, who I used to be, the capacities, knowledge and memories I once had. I grieve for the lost memories and knowledge, the lost places of my past I can no longer recall and that often cause me to feel disconnected from myself and from the family and friends I do still have close relationships with.

The homesickness for a home to which I cannot return, a home which maybe never was; the nostalgia, the yearning, the grief for the lost places of my past... This all relates to my experience of living with a diagnosis of dementia, and the fact that I can never return to being the person I once was, nor regain the knowledge and memories I have lost.

Richard Taylor said in conversations and in many of his presentations, 'You are not any closer to death than you were the day before you were diagnosed.' I absolutely agree with him, and often say 'We are all born with a death sentence.' However, being told I had dementia really was like a pseudo-death, and with death comes grief. You really do not have a choice.

The topics of grief and death and dying are closely connected to dementia, as although most of the dementias are recognised as terminal illnesses, and the discourse of dementia is 'sold' to us as a horrific, hideous, devastating disease to have, we are not given adequate grief counselling, if any at all. We are given support to get our end-of-life affairs in order, to get acquainted with aged care and, in my case and the cases of many others with dementia who I have spoken to around the world, very little else. We are Prescribed Disengagement®, a term I discuss in detail in Chapter 16.

This chapter is about the grief I have experienced, not all due to dementia, and a précis of what grief is. It is also about my thoughts and ideas of death and dying in general. I do recommend more of a focus is given to the experience of grief and dementia, and in the latter half of 2014 attended two seminars on the topic, the first I had heard of since being diagnosed, so I am hopeful the industry is taking more notice of the impact of dementia and the complicated grief that comes with the diagnosis.

When I think about my own experiences of grief, it seems that just when you think you are accepting an illness or a loss, your mind gives in to it again and throws you right back into the pit of grief, the sense of knowing what you are losing. It is often one step forward and then many steps backwards as you relive the intensity and anticipation of the loss caused through death of a loved one, or chronic and terminal illness.

After the initial shock and severe emotional pain experienced with a new grief comes the need for help, although this is often not recognised. In the very beginning there is always a shoulder to lean on and to cry on and a helping hand. It is there for the first few days and sometimes even weeks after the diagnosis. Then it disappears. For others, their lives go on as if nothing is happening, whilst your life is crumbling down around you. This is normal, and it is okay. Your judgements are impaired; your relationships are under strain due to the constancy of your illness or grief. Your new life brings with it permanent aching and longing for what once was, and your general sense of wellbeing has the potential to completely disappear. The sense of emptiness in your own life and on occasion towards your friends is off-putting to them, and unbearable to you. Life sometimes seems void.

Life with dementia can sometimes seem very hollow. The idea of not knowing your loved ones or even yourself in a mirror is daunting. Losing knowledge or even a sense of your own personal history and own identity is stressful.

I've heard Aboriginal Australians speaking about how their present is so connected to their past, with phrases like 'All my histories are through my past'. The impact on our personal and individual identity through the loss of memories is significant, and the impact on the grief even greater. If we can't remember our own past, what does that leave us with? Of course, we can live in the now, and I always try to do that anyway, but what happens when you also forget that? Living without memories, including knowledge and simple things like the spelling of or meanings of words, is much more difficult than anyone without memory loss could ever imagine.

My life has often been so full of tragedy it has sometimes been hard to breathe. Thirty years ago, a man I loved took his own life. He was 35 years old, a successful doctor with a brilliant career and a life full of friends and family. I was 27. Yet most of his achievements seemed unreal and senseless to him as he could never get rid of the intense burning pain inside his heart and soul…so much agony he could no longer go on. He was living with bipolar disorder and schizophrenia and could no longer see his way to continue living with them. Other aspects of my life have also brought profound grief, although rarely have I talked about it, usually acknowledged only to myself and in my personal writings.

Some time after David's death, I started writing as a way of expressing my pain, my lost love, and as a way to heal my grief following his death. More and more I have begun to question whether I had a choice about the grieving, whether I could have stopped it, or whether the grief itself was a disAbility. This particular voyage of grief was full of anguish and sorrow, but also one of great growth and new joy. In many ways, his death was the greatest gift he ever gave me, a rare jewel constantly prompting me to look within, to take life by the throat and never give up. Of course, it took me many years to make sense of his death, to be able to accept it as a major positive contribution to my own life and personal growth but I am certainly very relieved now that I have been able to see it like that.

Perhaps I could have made a choice about whether I allowed the grief and sadness to consume me for the first year or so after his death, but the grief was very real and in retrospect it lasted much longer than I realised and I feel sure is the reason I made a few poor major decisions in the first few years after his death. Ultimately volunteering for the Bereaved Through Suicide Support Group Inc. was my way of making sense of his death, but for a while it also allowed me to wallow in my wretchedness, too afraid to heal in case the healing would denigrate not only his life but my love for him. At times the wallowing allowed me to excuse myself from life, to excuse myself for not fulfilling my dreams and goals. It was a very acceptable cop-out, and one that no-one would dare deny my right to!

It often felt like it would be easy to give in and live with the sadness forever, and to never accept the new me or the changes to my world that took place after his death, and which I was forced to live in afterwards. It is very difficult to get used to living without someone you still love, and to get used to your new life without them.

This grief forced me to look inside my own heart, to accept my dark side, to delve into my own life more deeply than I had ever planned or thought I needed to, and to stop using my past as an excuse for not living life to the full. It helped me turn other negative experiences into inner strengths and to further develop my already well-developed resilience. It helped me to whole-heartedly embrace new experiences, even bad ones, to welcome them rather than reject them. Grief and loss is a large part of what has helped me become the person I am today and I am happy with who I am. It has taken me along many different paths, several of them tainted with the pain of loss and sadness. Life has offered itself to me with no boundaries, and I have had to make a choice to survive and grow and heal through each extraordinary event.

Grief is not something we can prepare for, nor compare. For a child, losing a teddy can be just as devastating (to the child) as an adult losing a wife or husband. The truth is, grief is selfish, in the sense that it is about 'self' – your own feelings and your personal feelings of loss. It has to be; you cannot experience the grief someone else feels. Perhaps having a similar loss is as close as you get, and this is why grief support groups work so well. To spend time with someone else who has lost a baby to Sudden Infant Death Syndrome (SIDS), or a partner or child to suicide, is very comforting and helps you normalise your own feelings. Our cells also have a grief memory, and so each time there is a new loss, our cells remember, a reason why someone may appear to be 'over-reacting' to a loss that others cannot see as significant.

In the last few years, my husband and I have experienced the sadness of a large number of deaths of many friends with younger onset dementia. We attend their funerals and mourn their loss, and where possible support the family and friends, and each other as best we can. However, this constant revisiting of grief, and of the death of friends with the same terminal illness as me, is extremely confronting, and it seems I am constantly experiencing a deepening grief, and it can sometimes feel like a deafening fear of what is ahead. I always have to ride the storm brewing inside of me.

Grief has many times felt like a constant companion, but now with dementia grief it virtually never goes away. When you lose someone you love, eventually, you learn to live without them, but you do heal, and change, and eventually you get used to your life without that person or thing.

Dementia grief is not like that, and can be extremely crippling; just as you get used to the loss of some function or capacity, it then gets worse, or you 'lose' some other function or capacity. Every time I decide I need to use a calculator, I then either realise through trying and failing that I can no longer work out how to, or I remember I can't, and then get consumed with guilt for needing to ask my husband, and a renewed sense of grief for the loss appears. This can happen hundreds of times a day, with things most people don't see or know about. It is often only when my husband is home for a whole day that even he sees how many things I can no longer do. Of course, I do still achieve a lot, and live a good life, but the grief of my losses, caused by the deterioration of current capacity, or of a new symptom of dementia, sits inside my heart and does not go away. It doesn't heal either, because I know things will get worse not better.

People with dementia have to be careful not to let the grief consume them constantly, and I believe we have to find ways to move through it and continue to live good lives, in spite of the complicated and ongoing process. We have to find ways to ignore it or put it on hold so that we, and not just our care partners, still live with joy in our hearts, and blogging and writing, especially poetry, has done that for me. That needs to start with those professionals supporting us recognising we have grief, and not just our care partners, and offering us professional grief support, not just counselling for the 'changes' that are ahead and being told to get our end-of-life affairs in order – support that is very often based around 'changes to behaviour' that may surface, squarely placing all of the 'changes' onto our shoulders, almost as if they are our fault.

Elisabeth Kubler-Ross said the stages of grief are denial, anger, bargaining, depression and acceptance. As far as dementia is concerned I have been through them all, and accepted it. There is also the sadness, and with dementia, the fear of your own future and of another loss of function or capacity. And then every time a new symptom appears or worsens, grief, sadness and more fear has the potential to reappear. As one of my blog readers said in a comment, there cannot be grief unless there has been love, or some sort of ownership of something within a relationship; ownership of our own functions is of course natural, and so the grief of losing them is profound. I try to be gentle on myself and those around me when I am feeling deep grief, but cannot always promise that.

The effect of my own grief since being diagnosed with dementia often means my energy and paddling has not been able to keep up with finding the ideas to write or edit many my own blogs, or even to speak clearly on some days. My blog draft folder remains very full, and completing any is difficult, and so when blogging I've 'cheated' on many days, 'borrowing' or reposting blogs, poems or YouTube clips that I felt still have some relevance, value and meaning. Writing a poem works well for me, as I can get away with fewer words, and yet still post my own writings. Writing poetry also helps me with healing and grief, and I have run some poetry writing workshops the last couple of years for people bereaved through suicide, who have also told me they have found it incredibly therapeutic.

Grieving for the loss of loved ones brings added pressure to the symptoms of dementia, or in fact, any other aspect of your life, with or without dementia. During the moments that sadness or tears overwhelm you, it is very difficult to think about anything else, and I've had to practise my advice given over the years to others when I was running the Bereaved Through Suicide Support Group. I sit in my garden a lot, regardless of the weather, and listen to music that is soothing, or meditate. The emptiness in my heart does not easily disappear. Knowing someone is in a better place, when considering how sick they had become, does not stop us from missing them and wishing they were still here. But knowing your own capacity and functioning is worsening, and will not ever get better, is most definitely challenging and brings with it a very complicated grief.

With dementia, I miss the capacity and memories I have lost, every single day.

Grief seems so selfish, and yet it needs to be. It is not selfish in a negative or indulgent way, it is our feelings of sadness centred on our self, and the only way we can properly deal with the feelings of sadness and loss. The energy required living with and working through grief is high, and definitely affects the paddling needed to manage the symptoms of dementia. Many days I have not even bothered to try to hide them, just giving in to the grief I have felt. This is the right thing to do, and I realise there are still many days ahead like this.

One friend overseas reminded me how lucky I am to have my soul mate to grieve with me, to be by my side. The loneliness of being home alone to deal with grief can make it more difficult; it somehow exacerbates sadness, yet time alone is often when we do our best grieving and I know that when David died, I spent most of the time alone for some time afterwards as it was too emotionally difficult to be with people who were not grieving for him. But to have someone to hold onto and hug, when the going gets tough is truly a gift, especially if they just allow you to grieve in your own way.

Grief is a journey through darkness, affecting every aspect of your living and functioning, but it is worth reminding ourselves…it can also be a path towards a brighter light and a much deeper understanding of life and self. The darkest dark never put out the dimmest candle.

Grief and loss can bring people closer, or tear them apart, and I have seen it both ways.

No matter how hard we try to let go of it, grief follows us around wherever we go. New grief reignites or reminds us of old losses, and if we have had previous significant losses, then we have to work harder to adjust to a new one.

Times like Christmas and other significant occasions like birthdays and anniversaries usually throw the newly bereaved into total turmoil. The 'first times' without them at the table for something like Christmas is really difficult to adjust to, and usually heightens our sense of loss.

And yet, death gives life meaning. It creates the contrast, and finally offers the reality of who we really are. These days, very few will worry about burning in hell, some might still fear death, but many of us are now worrying about dying. '*Why?*' you may ask. Most doctors have witnessed patients die undignified, soulless, high-tech deaths and hoped for something better for themselves and their patients. Most of us now have watched the same horrific and inhumane tragedy. But what does a good death look like and how high a priority should it be for health services?

If death is defeat, then it won't be a high priority. But if *a good death is the conclusion of a good life* then it has to be a priority.

We have watched a number of family members and friends die the last few years. They were at varying ages; some were *dying* not so much from disease than from old age, but many younger friends were dying from dementia, which happens to cause many of the same symptoms as old age. None of them were in acute medical states. All of them were in bodies that were shutting down. What is becoming clear to me about a good death is that one size won't fit all. We want to be as different in dying as we are in living. Different cultures, times and religions have different concepts of a good death. Some want it sudden, some slow. Some want a quiet death with minimal medical involvement. Some want a lot of fanfare.

Others want to follow Dylan Thomas and *rage, rage against the dying of the light*, squeezing every last drop from life.

A few choose to kill themselves (suicide), while others would like to choose when they die (euthanasia). Even in countries that have legalised euthanasia very few people choose to die that way, suggesting that perhaps it's far less important than we want to believe. But pressure to legalise euthanasia seems likely to grow, combined with people wanting increasing choices on how they die. Personally, I am in favour of a person's right to take their own life if they are living with a terminal illness, including dementia. The issue with dementia is that we would have to action our desire, before we lose capacity, so even if the law changes in countries like Australia, it may not solve the problem of people with dementia who would choose euthanasia. It is a very complex issue.

I will share this simply to give context to the topic of euthanasia, one I believe many people have strong opinions on, either for or against. When I was studying for my undergraduate degree in Psychology, I chose euthanasia as a topic for one of my major essays. Before David took his own life, I agreed with euthanasia. After he died, I disagreed with euthanasia. Some years later I found my way to believing his suicide was, in his reality, euthanasia, due to his mental illness being like a 'cancer' inside his heart (brain), and found that more acceptable to live with. I was back to agreeing with euthanasia. Now, I am unsure, but I would not deny another person's right to it, and do believe the law should change on this.

It is clear that each individual's viewpoints on euthanasia will remain vehemently divided, based on one's personal philosophical, religious or other beliefs and experiences. It is evident that physician-assisted death is already occurring with the use of pain-relieving drugs which speed up the process of death all around the world. What right do we have to impose our religious, philosophical or personal views onto another individual? The biggest debate will surely be the one for non-voluntary assisted suicide due to the implications of its possible abuse by physicians, hospital staff or family members. We could also say voluntary euthanasia is happening in ways we currently term suicide.

The one thing I do know quite a lot about is suicide grief, and after my essay at university exploring euthanasia, my one concern remains about what the grief could be like for those family and friends who do not agree with euthanasia; it might be like suicide grief, which is truly devastating.

The term euthanasia versus assisted or voluntary suicide has explosive implications on the loved ones left behind to grieve, and the possible effect of suicide grief rather than grief associated with other death. As the term euthanasia implies, it is a very fine line between it being a more acceptable death or a suicide death.

There was nothing in the literature at the time on the impact of grief following euthanasia, and I think that topic deserves some energy and focus. Grief and loss, I believe, is far more important than most of us would believe, and regardless of our human right to make a choice, we have some responsibility when we are thinking about euthanasia to consider those people our death would impact. It is not only a religious or personal choice.

One might also wonder, is death the ultimate form of consumer resistance, consumer choice?

As the baby boomers turn their thoughts to death they are unlikely to accept the squalid end that may happen in a health service almost completely preoccupied with life at the expense of death.

The diagnosis of dying is one of the most crucial that a doctor must make. It is one of the most difficult we will ever receive. Research shows that doctors consistently overestimate the time patients have left to live. In order to help patients to a good death doctors must readjust themselves, recognising that death is closer than they think, and usually closer than the dying person wants.

We must recalibrate ourselves and accept also that a death of a loved one is almost always sooner than we would wish for. And more than that, we must learn to celebrate their lives, and our relationships, together as one, with as much love as possible, before they die.

For families who have Mr Dementia sitting at their Christmas table, or a loved one locked in a secure dementia unit missing out on sitting at the Christmas table, it can be more difficult than a deceased loved one not being there at all. Bob De Marco[1] wrote about his first Christmas without his mother Dotty who died in May 2012 from dementia of the Alzheimer's type: 'I am a little sad and a little lonely. But, the sadness is more than trumped by all the happy memories.'

For me, spending time with lots of family or old friends is more challenging, as there is usually a constant phrase in the conversations as so many sentences began with 'Remember when...' and on the occasions when I can remember an event or conversation, it is great.

But at the times I cannot remember, it is lonely, and on the inside of my heart, it increases the grief and sadness, and the fear and feelings of isolation.

It is easier to pretend to remember, but not always then as easy then to participate in extended conversations about events and people, as pretending only works at the very beginning. This is when the feelings of humiliation and embarrassment enter the inner world of the person with dementia, even if they say nothing about it. By blogging, I will be able to 'remember when' I thought or did something, and with the love and support of my immediate family and a few close friends, for now I get through it.

For those of you who are experiencing the loss and grief of a new diagnosis of dementia, may you be surrounded by your family and close friends, by those who care for and love for you unconditionally, and who I hope will be there for you when you need to talk, not just when it suits them, and who will be silent with you, or cry with you, and also allow you to grieve in your own unique ways.

---

1   www.alzheimersreadingroom.com/2012/11/bob-demarco-founder-alzheimers-reading-room.html

We've all experienced grief. We've all felt those intense rolling waves of emotion. But do we all experience the same feelings each time we lose a loved one? Grief is hard work, and it is lonely, and it impacts those of us living with dementia greatly.

What are the stages of grief?

Many have tried to explain what grief is; some have even identified certain stages of grief. Probably the most well-known of these might be from *Elizabeth Kubler-Ross's* book, *On Death and Dying* (1969). In it, she identified five stages that a dying patient experiences when informed of their terminal prognosis.

The stages Kubler-Ross identified are:

- Denial (This isn't *happening* to me!).

- Anger (Why is this happening to *me*?).

- Bargaining (If I do this, I won't die…or I promise I'll be a better person *if…*).

- Depression (I don't *care* any more).

- Acceptance (*I'm ready* for whatever comes).

Many people believe that these stages of grief are also experienced by others when they have lost a loved one. Personally, I think of these definitions as emotional reactions or behaviours rather than stages, per se. I believe we may certainly experience some of them. But, I believe, just as strongly, that there is no script for grief; that we cannot expect to feel any of our emotions in a particular set pattern. I do agree that acceptance is probably the last emotion felt, and in some instances it may be the only one. For some, acceptance never comes.

A lesser known definition of the stages of grief is described by *Dr Roberta Temes* in the book, *Living with an Empty Chair: A Guide Through Grief* (1992). Temes describes three particular types of behaviour exhibited by those experiencing grief and loss. They are:

- Numbness (mechanical functioning and social insulation).

- Disorganisation (intensely painful feelings of loss).

- Reorganisation (re-entry into a more 'normal' social life).

I am better able to relate to this definition as it seems to more accurately reflect the types of feelings I have experienced and observed. Within these types of behaviours might well be most of the feelings described in Kubler-Ross's writings as well.

Which list is the best one?

Perhaps both of these lists, and many others that we may have seen, are all descriptive of some of the emotions and functions we go through when we lose a loved one.

Grief, like so many other things in our complex lives, can't be reduced to a neat list with absolute definitions, timelines, strategies, goals, and completion dates. If that were the case, it might be easier. Grief is as individual as those of us who feel it, and as varied as the circumstances of death or loss which occur.

Will I go through every stage of grief?

With the grief associated with dementia, probably not. Sorry. If a 98-year-old grandfather died in his sleep I think there would be different stages of grief and loss experienced than if a two-year-old child were run over by a car and killed. I experienced this with the death of an older aunt, killed in a hit-and-run accident. If a person has had a long life, death is somewhat expected as the natural scheme of things, but her life being cut short through a crime somehow made it less bearable.

There will always be emotions of grief and loss but they might be more for what *we* will miss. If for example, a life is cut short unexpectedly, there may well be feelings of denial, anger, bargaining, depression, grief about what they will miss by dying at a young age, but in most cases eventually there is likely to be acceptance.

Just as we have different emotional reactions to anything that happens in our lives, so too will we experience grief and loss in different ways. I think the important thing to remember is that there is a wide range of emotions that may be experienced; to expect to feel some of them and to know that we cannot completely control the process. I used to liken it to being at sea on a life raft, with no rudder and no say over what the weather was going to bring each day, and still find this analogy works for me. Dementia is also very much like that for me, as it also feels like I am drifting at sea on a rudderless boat, with very limited ability to stop any of the changes and losses ahead.

After a loss, do we ever stop grieving?

Grieving used to be much more ritualistic than it is today. In generations past there were set periods of time when certain customs must be observed:

- Widows wore all black clothing for one year and drab colours forever after.

- Mourners could not attend social gatherings for months.

- Laughter and gaiety were discouraged for weeks or months.

Today most of us are free from these restrictions and might even be confused about when we should be finished grieving.

In reality, we'll probably never be finished grieving, but we do eventually learn to live with loss and the changes to our world caused by loss. Dementia, however, brings a new dimension to grief, as the losses continue as capacity or functioning disappears, or deteriorates.

Most will never forget the person they grieve for, although a person with dementia might, and reminding us of a deceased loved one, friend or relative, if we have forgotten they have died, may be more traumatic than it is worth being totally honest about. Our feelings may be tempered more with good memories than sadness as time passes, but that isn't to say that waves of raw emotion won't overcome us long after we think we should be over grief.

I think the trick here is to understand that the feelings will occur, try to keep them in perspective, try to understand not so much why you feel a certain way, but to simply accept your feelings, and if there are any unresolved issues that cause particular emotional pain, forgive yourself and others, and give yourself time. If necessary talk with someone about it, including seeing a professional grief counsellor, or write (or type) about your feelings in a journal. I was taught by psychologist and friend Kevin Harvey about the value of keeping a daily diary of how I was feeling, and this not only helps you let go of emotional pain, it allows you to see progress, even on the darkest of days. With dementia, this can work in reverse, as it is easy to see the deterioration in functioning, but the value of writing about it, for me, does help to dissolve the pain of the individual losses. Richard Taylor reinforced the value of this for me.

There is no completion date to grieving…it is better to just let your emotions flow.

Loss and grief are a normal part of accepting a terminal illness. It is more often associated with death, and this can make the experience of loss in dementia even more difficult, as we don't accept or validate that what we are going through is in fact a grieving process. The dementia sector is only waking up to the grief component of dementia, and prior to 2014 I never heard it discussed, nor were we offered grief counselling following the diagnosis of dementia. This, I believe, does need to change.

Grief after a diagnosis of dementia is not very different to any other loss, and includes: shock and denial, fear, guilt and anger; it is normal to feel anger about what is happening, and in the early stages it is a big part of our grief. The big difference is, we are not going to recover, but instead will continue to deteriorate and then die.

It is important to help people with dementia find ways to overcome the anger and replace it with positive and meaningful life and positive thinking. Bargaining also takes place, for example if I do this, or take that, or I will get better, and is another normal part of grief. Depression can be a part of grief; it needs proper assessment; it may not need medication as it is also a 'normal' part of the grieving process; management through positive activity and counselling may be more productive.

Reflection also becomes a significant part of the grieving process. Loneliness (we feel very alone when first diagnosed) is a significant part of grief too, and is added to by the stigma of dementia. The trauma of anticipatory grief for future losses is also a significant and constant progression in the earlier stages as people with dementia slowly lose their abilities and often still have a lot of insight; there is a constant fear of *what function or skill will I lose next?* Many people with dementia will eventually find acceptance, the last stage of grief, although I suspect this is much harder for our loved ones to find as they watch on, suffering.

Having insight is vital to acceptance but, in the face of dementia, can be terrifying as, with insight, one must face up to what is ahead.

However, acceptance is the final stage of grief, and it is important to help the person with dementia and their family to get there. Like Viktor Frankl, I feel it is important for the person with dementia 'to bear witness to the uniquely human potential…which is to transform a personal tragedy into a triumph, to turn one's predicament into a human achievement' (2006).

Itzhak Perlman, the violinist who needs crutches to get on stage, said:[2] 'It is the artist's task to find out how much music you can still make with what you have left', and people with dementia have this same vital task to find their own 'art' or 'creativity' in their lived experience with dementia, if they possibly can. Like him we must struggle to cope, to create, to live our own unique lives, despite the limitations brought on by dementia. This is no easy feat, and is a constant battle, as it is unlike needing crutches for an unchanging disAbility. Our disAbilities are increasing and changing.

We can discover new talents, focusing on aspects of our lives such as relationships, emotions and spirituality, rather than being too focused on changing our cognition.

2   www.goodreads.com/author/quotes/6901.Itzhak_Perlman

By assigning dementia a secondary place, we have more potential to enhance these other aspects of our humanity. Basil Hume, when he was diagnosed with cancer, said, 'I have received two wonderful graces. First the time to prepare for a new future; Secondly, I find myself – uncharacteristically – at peace.' It is through finding meaning in life, even with a diagnosis of dementia, that it is possible to create a new sense of purpose and meaning, and importantly to overcome the intense fear of loss and death.

There will be new meaning to life, new ways of thinking to get used to, old ways to get used to losing, many questions never ever answered. New and raw grief leads us to want our old life back, our old happiness to return; it doesn't tell us we have to get used to a new way of thinking and living, it doesn't even hint at the prospect of healing. It feels like it will never go away, never get better, and never let us smile again. And yet, the sun will always keep rising, the sky will still be blue and our power to heal each other can still be fuelled by love.

I have always had a penchant for helping others, particularly when bereaved, in part fuelled by my great-grandmother, grandmother and an aunt, and in part fuelled by my own losses. The following is part of an email my amazingly loving and supportive husband sent to me in 2011 when we were facing the death of another friend:

Subject: A note from the heart.

To my dear wife, You are the only person I know who gives of herself without some form of hidden agenda. You are thoughtful and caring. You are involved in life and supporting others more than anybody has the right to ask, but I know you wouldn't have it any other way. I hope things are not too hard on you this morning as I know how close to the bone all of this is cutting. Your absolute number one fan. Love you forever and a bit. Peter.

Why would I not want to continue to share the burdens and wounds of others, especially with that amount of love and support behind me? Our love, and his understanding and encouragement make it so much easier. And I love supporting others through grief and loss; it has been one of the most meaningful things I have ever done in my own life. It is a huge part of who I am, and why I advocate so strongly for others also living with a dementia.

Death and dying is a part of life, and the bonus of being given the possibility of a more finite time to live is that it does make you think very deeply about your own life. Yes, I do believe it is a bonus as it helps us live more deeply, to live every day as if it is our last, just in case it is. It has also helped my husband and I seek to only see the good in each other, and to let go of the petty disagreements, almost always there only because of one's individual need to be 'right'.

With the diagnosis of a terminal illness, including dementia, mortality gets to sit at your table, right next to the knife and fork, up close and personal, whispering messages that you might die much sooner than you thought. You do not get to continue to view death from the large platform called life, but from the edge of the stage, just behind the curtain, as if waiting for your cue to die. A diagnosis of a terminal illness makes you feel temporary, transient, and somehow perishable; mortal. Facing up to the fact that dementia is a terminal illness is made more difficult because of the focus being more on the thought of your own quality of life being compromised, of not living fully functionally, until you die, and the thought of not being in a position to make your own choices. The notion of not knowing your loved ones, or not remembering yourself in a mirror, makes it very daunting, and colours the reality of the illness, making it hard to make end-of-life decisions in a timely fashion.

Aside from terminal illness, events such as 9/11 or war or natural disasters like floods, tsunamis, earthquakes and landslides can bring you close to facing death, but only if you are 'in' the experience, rather than just watching them from afar via the radio or television, as if they are merely a distant visitor to your life and not close up on your own stage. The positive impact of events like these, and terminal illnesses including dementia, is that once the shock and anger subsides, your view of the world and yourself changes, and lights come on inside your tunnel that didn't show up before. There is a type of freedom missing previously, and clarity of thought and insight. And a deeper love and laughter that, although sometimes tinged with sadness, can set you free.

Dying is what is ahead of all of us, whether it is from dementia, cancer, or some other disease, or just an ageing and failing body. Being born is a death sentence. Living well is optional though, and I believe we need to make a choice eventually to have a good time while we are alive, or we might as well be dead anyway.

My great-grandmother (Gran) used to say, 'You should cry at a wedding, and be happy at a funeral', her wisdom coming from her strong Christian faith, but also her belief that your real troubles start when you marry or get into a permanent relationship, and are over when you die! Gran and my maternal grandmother (nanny), both deceased many years ago, and my aunts, two of whom are thankfully still alive, have impacted my thinking greatly and are still my mentors to this day. I love these strong, compassionate women who love me or loved me no matter what, and who have guided me through life, even if they do not realise how much they have done so.

We all live until we die and I salute them for their openness and honesty with me about life, and about death.

The lessons I continue to learn from illness, death and dying, and the impacts of loss and grief never cease to astound and surprise me.

CHAPTER 13

The Emotional Toll of Letting Go

LOVE AND LETTING GO

As we sit and watch
The one we love in the last stages of dying
The hardest thing to say is
"It is OK to let go"

Let go and move on
Find your freedom in the next world
I will be here
You will be there

But you will never be forgotten
Take your last breath
Freely
And in that, your last breath

I will breathe in
And make it my own
We will always be
Together forever

DEDICATED TO MICHAEL AND GREGORY

(KATE SWAFFER 2015)

In a blog comment some time ago about me handing things over to my husband or BUB (Back-Up Brain), I responded with this: 'I have had to give up a couple of things this week, and hand the responsibility over to Pete.' I felt and still feel physically *sick* when I have to hand over something I can no longer do, and incompetent, and guilty and ashamed, and embarrassed and humiliated. Regardless of the fact I know he does not mind at all. The more I thought about it, the more I know it was an important topic for this book as I suspect many people with dementia feel these things.

As I asked my husband to take over, the physical response was instant, and stayed with me as a vague nausea for some time, and returns now whenever I think about it. Prior to one of the visits to my neurologist, I had typed up a list of things to discuss, having had my husband review and add to it, in an effort not to forget things when we went in. On the day, my speech was not brilliant, and so I handed this job of communicating with the specialist over to my BUB. He needed a very strong reinforcement that it was okay for him to take over and in fact not what I wanted, but what I needed. He looked vaguely distressed about it too, as this was new to him. He probably felt physically sick about it too. He has said that sometimes, when a symptom becomes noticeably worse, or a new one appears, he feels like he has been kicked in the stomach. I know the few times I have not been able to recall his name we have both been devastated. It is, quite simply, traumatic for us both.

More recently, and definitely since the first manuscript of this book was sent to my publishers, I have noticed my ability to find the names of things and people has become significantly worse; once again, this brings on the physical feelings of wanting to vomit as I reel against the tide of changes and work my way through the emotions of even more losses. It does usually subside, at least until the next time...

I have had to accept help from family and friends for transport for years now, but still feel like I am a burden, even when reassured I am not. It still makes me feel guilty asking for others to pick me up. There are quite a few other areas where I have had to relinquish things and accept assistance, like the Webster packs to manage my medication. Each one sounds simple, and helpful. And they are. But if I group or list them together collectively, they start to add up to quite a list, even though to an onlooker I am still functioning in so many areas.

The only way I have been able to cope is to see them as disAbilities, which also empowers me to rise above them, and then I've had to see all of these supports as 'life enhancement aids', or they would continue to bring me unstuck emotionally.

The fear of losing a function or ability is powerful, and has helped me fight against the symptoms of dementia, has helped me stay motivated to treat them as disAbilities. But as the disAbilities worsen, and I need assistance or the help of someone else taking over, the fear the ability will not come back is reinforced. The grief is heightened by this fear, and sometimes anger or anxiety, and the denial bubble bursts with a resounding bang! I feel guilt for being a burden, even though my husband reassures me I am not, and he is there for me, and wants to help. In fact he says, he wants to help, whenever I need it. And I believe him. I know I would feel the same, but this knowledge does not easily remove my burden of guilt.

My husband and I are in it together, I know this 100 per cent, and believe it 100 per cent. I know I would do exactly the same for him, or my children or best friends or other loved ones. I just never thought about needing this kind of help myself. Having nursed, and been a mother and a volunteer, I have always helped others, and I find it very challenging to hold out my own hand, and ask for and then actually accept help. Self-love allows me to feel worthy of the help (thankfully), but still does not stop me from wanting to object, or quite often from refusing to ask for help! I have often advocated for the rights of those groups of people who are marginalised or less well off than me, and it is emotionally challenging and sometimes distressing to put myself in that same category.

It is human nature to become too attached to things or people. And it can be very difficult to find ways to let go of these attachments even if we know that they are not good for us. I wonder, though, is being attached to our own ability to function wrong?

One of the first things to do in letting go is to have a good hard look at the thing/s you are letting go of; are they really that good for us? For the person with dementia, it is not easy to believe losing something like the ability to recall or remember something or someone, or how to get dressed or make a cup of tea, is not valuable to our life.

Facing the strange emptiness caused by the loss of a physical or cognitive function is extremely difficult, not at all like giving up cigarettes or eating too much fatty food.

One of the best ways I have found to help with the pain of letting go of something is to wrap yourself in love and laughter; find family, friends, or other people to love and support you. And also to spend time with others who have a diagnosis of a dementia, in a support group exclusive to us, where we do not have to feel ashamed, embarrassed, nor explain anything. Dementia Alliance International offers this, which I will extrapolate on later in this book. I am ever grateful for my wonderfully supportive husband, children, special friends and my global dementia community. I'm also very thankful for an innate sense of humour, which has apparently become funnier since Mr Dementia, or Larry, as dementia is laughingly referred to in my house, arrived!

CHAPTER 14

Myths of Dementia

Roland Barthes wrote, in 1957, 'Myth is neither a lie nor a confession: it is an inflexion.' In that sense, therefore, a myth is a modulation of the voice or a change in the form of a word, usually modification or affixation, signalling change in such grammatical functions as tense, voice, mood, person, gender, number, or case. In a sense, it is an angle or a bend.

The late Dr Richard Taylor[1] was a person living beyond the symptoms of dementia, probably of the Alzheimer's type, and he and I gave separate presentations on the *Myths of Dementia* during Dementia Awareness Month 2014, as part of the Dementia Alliance International (DAI) programme. Both are available on the DAI YouTube.[2] He was not a physician but a Clinical Psychologist. He said he had become through his own research and life 'a reluctant expert of living with dementia'. We would both always encourage you to discuss the myths of dementia with your physician, and draw your own conclusions based upon your own research and life and the advice of professionals. He was a mentor and very good friend to me, someone who I have often looked to for wisdom and inspiration. He

----

1　www.richardtaylorphd.com
2　www.youtube.com/channel/UC9OU-TO5MmvYPhmz6j7DYlg?sub_ confirmation=1

regularly reminded me to decide for myself or others will decide for me.

This chapter is a précis of the notes from two different presentations we separately gave on our experience of the myths of dementia.

Richard presented on Roland Barthes's many contributions to philosophy, collected in his book *Mythologies* (1957). Barthes frequently interrogated specific cultural materials in order to expose how bourgeois society asserted its values through them. For example, the portrayal of wine in French society as a robust and healthy habit is a bourgeois ideal that is contradicted by certain realities (that is, that wine can be unhealthy and inebriating). He found semiotics, the study of signs, useful in these interrogations. Barthes explained that these bourgeois cultural myths were 'second-order signs' or 'connotations'. For example, a picture of a full, dark bottle is a signifier that relates to a specific signified: a fermented, alcoholic beverage. However, the bourgeoisie relate it to a new signified: the idea of healthy, robust, relaxing experience. Motivations for such manipulations vary, from a desire to sell products to a simple desire to maintain the status quo.

I felt, in the context of dementia, this was very interesting, as the myths of dementia have been hard to dispel, so let's first look at the definition of a myth:

1 A traditional or legendary story, usually concerning some being or hero or event, with or without a determinable basis of fact or a natural explanation, especially one that is concerned with deities or demigods and explains some practice, rite or phenomenon of nature.

2 Stories or matter of this kind: realm of myth.

3   Any invented story, idea, or concept.

4   An imaginary or fictitious thing or person.

5   An unproved or false collective belief that is used to justify a social institution.

The word 'myth' comes from the French *mythe*, and directly from the Modern Latin *mythus*, from the Greek *mythos*, meaning 'speech, thought, story, myth, anything delivered by word of mouth, of unknown origin'; a fable or a word (Etymonline, Online Etymology Dictionary).

Myths are 'stories about divine beings, generally arranged in a coherent system; they are revered as true and sacred; they are endorsed by rulers and priests; and closely linked to religion. Once this link is broken, and the actors in the story are not regarded as gods but as human heroes, giants or fairies, it is no longer a myth but a folktale. Where the central actor is divine but the story is trivial...the result is religious legend, not myth' (Simpson and Rond 2000, p.254). The general sense of it being described as an 'untrue story, rumor' dates from 1840.

Personally I believe the fifth definition of myth – *an unproved or false collective belief that is used to justify a social institution* – is being held onto by our health and aged care system.

Why? I think so that they can *justify their position of power over people with dementia*, allowing those running the government and health care system to justify it as appropriate and 'their duty of care' to completely ignore many of our most basic human rights, such as restraining us physically and chemically, and not providing us with more ethical pathways of post-diagnostic support.

No-one with mental illness is automatically locked up for their own good, and yet the frail elderly and people with dementia are locked up all the time. The myths support the continued bent of restraint with drugs or physical restraints and the 'do no harm' ethos has been twisted to 'restraint or tracking is being used so they [people with dementia] don't come to harm'. It is a cop-out, and in my humble opinion needs desperately to change as without change we will never ever receive person- or relationship-centred care.

There are probably hundreds of myths about a diagnosis of dementia, and this chapter seeks to explore a few of them.

Popular myths of dementia

There is no point diagnosing dementia as nothing can be done, and there is no cure.

I see significant value in an early diagnosis, regardless of the fact there is no cure and treatment of any kind for less than half of those diagnosed with dementia, and will discuss why later on. This is not based so much on having the capacity to ensure your end-of-life wishes are in order, but allows you to take control of your health, and work on positive psychosocial and non-pharmacological interventions such as improving your health, exercise, and so on.

Dementia is a normal part of ageing.

Alzheimer's disease and other dementias are not a part of normal ageing. Almost 40 per cent of people over the age of 65 experience some form of memory loss. When there is no underlying medical condition causing this memory loss, it is known as 'age-associated memory impairment', which is considered a part of the normal ageing process.

But brain diseases like Alzheimer's and other dementias are different.

Age-associated memory impairment and dementia can be told apart in a number of ways. In general, a memory problem may become a concern if it begins to affect your day-to-day living. Older adults do not go on to develop Alzheimer's disease or other dementia as a normal part of ageing. It's important to know when to see your doctor about memory concerns but it's equally important to know that forgetting someone's name doesn't necessarily mean that you are getting dementia.

We are 'fading away' and 'not all there'.
Even though we may be changing, we are always still all there. A person dying from terminal cancer or motor neurone disease is all there, and so are people with dementia. We change each and every day, and after every significant experience, and it is no different for people with dementia. As a friend and colleague of mine John Sandblom,[3] Board member and co-founder of Dementia Alliance International, once said:

> *We are just changing in ways the rest of you aren't, we have increasing disabilities and the sooner it is looked at that way instead of the stigmas, misunderstandings and complete lies, the better for all of us living with dementia. We desperately need others to enable us, not further disable us!*

We can't communicate with you.
Even in the later stages of dementia, when some people lose the ability to speak, they [we] can still communicate – if only others would take the time to watch and listen to the non-verbal signs of communication. When I was volunteering in a low-care residential care home a few years ago, a lady with advanced dementia decided to tag along with my father-in-law and me. The staff regularly told me not to waste my time with her, as she could no longer speak. However, I took a real shine to her, and had time to spend

3   www.earlyonsetatypicalalzheimers.com/blog

with her, so two to three times a week we either sat or walked together, arm in arm. Initially she would ask me if she knew me, with a worried look on her face. Over the course of a few months, she not only recognised my face and started greeting me with a smile, but she shared with me all sorts of things about herself, where she had grown up, how her father had the first car in her district, and other interesting details of her life. Yes, she could talk – she just needed people to take the time for her to find her words, and then for them to listen. Each time I would meet with her, I would tell her the things she had last shared with me, and she would eventually be delighted that she had thought there was nothing in there (pointing to her head!), she still knew these things about herself, and 'wished others would take time to let her find her words'. Her words, not mine.

Another lady, when I worked in a dementia unit in 1977, ironically the first dementia-specific unit in Adelaide, where the staff there also told me she was mute, started speaking to me in the toilet one day. When I asked her why she wouldn't speak to the other staff, she said, 'it is because they treat me as if I am stupid'. Her words, not mine.

This is the analogy I use for better supporting people with memory loss or word-finding difficulties: *For the memory impaired, memory is like a stack of china.* For me, this is why it is important to give people with dementia time to collect what is left of their thoughts, and the time to find the words to tell you about them. It seems crucial to me that you resist the urge to give us a nudge to hurry us along as that will most likely make us stumble and lose our footing – our words – and this is when our 'plates' come crashing down.

My point being, of course, if you give us time, it is quite likely we will find a way to communicate with you.

*We don't have memory loss therefore we
can't possibly have dementia.*

Many people become forgetful as they become older. This
is common and is often not due to dementia. There are
also other disorders such as depression and an underactive
thyroid that can cause memory problems. Dementia is the
most serious form of memory problem. It causes a loss
of mental ability, and other symptoms. Dementia can be
caused by various disorders which affect parts of the brain
involved with thought processes. Most cases are caused by
Alzheimer's disease, vascular dementia, or dementia with
Lewy bodies. Symptoms of dementia develop gradually
and typically become worse over a number of years. There
are many dementias where the person does not experience
any, or very little memory loss until the late stages of the
disease process, although because of the activities such as
memory walks or memory cafes, most people think if there
is no apparent memory loss, then the person cannot have
dementia, which is wrong.

*We can still speak and function in public
therefore we can't have dementia.*

This is a common misperception or myth, especially for
those of us diagnosed early in our disease. Just because
we can still speak, and appear in the 30 minutes someone
spends with us to be functioning well, does not mean we
don't have dementia. The analogy of the swan, calm and
serene on the surface, paddling below the surface to stay
afloat, is very apt. And then there are many of us who have
support from someone at home, and use laminated lists and
other memory or function supports that others never see.

My husband sees that sometimes I cannot remember
what something is called, and these days, even sometimes

his name, but by using generic language more often, I can still get away with appearing to be fully functional. I always use notes now as well, especially when I am being interviewed or presenting, although the notes are working less well due to being less able to follow them now as my disAbilities relating to reading are changing.

Many people with dementia appear to be functioning well, even though they have increasing disAbilities, and the more we learn to manage the disAbilities, I believe *for many*, the longer we will function independently and well. The late Dr Richard Taylor in the USA, Christine Bryden in Australia, Agnes Houston in Scotland, Peter Ashley in the UK, Helga Rohra in Germany, Jennifer Bute in the UK, and many others who have been diagnosed for a much longer time than me, are still appearing to function well, even though I know for many of them the symptoms are increasing, and our abilities are deteriorating.

We don't look like we have dementia.
Quite frankly, what is someone with dementia supposed to look like?! Unlike a person born with Down's syndrome, we don't develop features that indicate dementia, and we are very rarely diagnosed at end stage, when it may be more obvious that we have a dementia. A couple of years ago, a psychologist said to me in a public forum, 'You don't look like you have dementia'. After years of being offended by being told I am lying about the diagnosis, or whatever other insulting comments have been made (and there have literally been hundreds, also experienced by many others living with a dementia), I replied, 'and you don't look like an arsehole!' No-one argues or makes claims of lying to a person doing well with cancer or any other terminal illness, so why is it so hard for people to believe we can (and do) do well with

dementia? It is indeed a continuing conundrum. Almost never is a person diagnosed at the end stage of any disease, including dementia.

We don't feel pain.
There is a growing body of research that has found that many of the symptoms often written off as 'just a part of the challenging behaviours of dementia' – agitation, aggression, withdrawal or repeatedly asking for attention – are actually untreated pain.

According to a recent review in the journal *Clinical Intervention in Ageing,* pain is the biggest cause of such symptoms – including language breakdown. However, the authors concluded that while pain is often the underlying cause of some behaviour, patients may be given 'inappropriate' sedating medication instead.

It's not that dementia itself causes pain, but the 47.5 million people in the world with dementia tend to be older and therefore more prone to aches and pains. Many patients lose the ability to talk, but even those who are coherent may struggle to find the right words to describe their discomfort.

The problem is that not all health professionals or care partners are yet aware of this, so they dismiss changes to behaviour such as becoming agitated as part of dementia, says Pat Schofield, professor of nursing at the University of Greenwich.

Historically, we used to believe that people with dementia do not feel pain because of the effects that their illness has on the brain but in recent years we realised that is not so; they are just as likely to experience pain but they cannot express it.

Think how frustrating that must be – you can't find the words to tell someone, 'I'm in agony' or 'This is hurting'.

Just like everyone else, of course people with dementia feel physical and emotional pain. We are, after all, still human beings…

People can't live beyond a diagnosis of dementia.
Living well at any time of our life is probably what everyone wants, but add in the diagnosis of dementia, and the Prescribed Disengagement®, and many of us think we can no longer live well. It is possible, and although working hard supporting ourselves with non-pharmacological interventions, and on remaining positive and meaningfully engaged, is not a cure, it does improve our quality of life and wellbeing. There is a growing body of research to support this, and as we are most likely further away from a cure than we were ten years ago, it is imperative we strive to live as well as we can. I call it the Olympics of my life, and although I am terrified of the day when I will no longer be independently functional, for now, it has increased my sense of wellbeing. Living well, however, is a challenging term for many people with dementia, and in Chapter 16 I will discuss the notion of living beyond dementia further, but we desperately need the health care sector, and the community, not only to support us to die, but to support us to live beyond the diagnosis of a dementia, and as positively as humanly possible.

We know how to 'cure' Alzheimer's or some other dementia…
all we need do is spend more money on research.
There is no cure for dementia and no medicine that will reverse it. However, there are some medicines that may be used to help slow down some types of dementia. Medication is generally used for different reasons. First, as treatment to help with symptoms that affect thinking and memory (cognitive symptoms); unfortunately many treatments are

used to modify 'challenging behaviours', when in fact what is needed is better education in understanding the needs of a person with dementia, as they usually stem from unmet needs or being unable to communicate in the same way as before. We need research on the non-pharmacological and positive psychosocial interventions for dementia to improve our wellbeing and quality of life, not just for a cure.

Alzheimer's disease is not dementia.
Of course Alzheimer's disease is a type of dementia. It is more correct to say, if diagnosed with any dementia, that you have a dementia, probably of this or that type. In the same way that the words 'fruit' or 'car' are umbrella terms, 'dementia' is an umbrella term for around 130 different types or causes of dementia.

Eat more of ****** *and you will be 'cured' or at least the progression of your symptoms will slow down.*
This works in favour of people and companies who, quite simply, probably only want to sell you a product of some kind. Sadly, people with dementia are often very vulnerable, and easy targets for people wanting to make money out of us. That is not to say that I don't agree with making an effort to improve our diet and our lifestyle, including doing cognitive and physical exercise and reducing isolation, as these are all known risk reduction factors for dementia and may also be found to slow the progression of the disease.

You can't 'live' with Alzheimer's disease, you can only die with and from it.
We are all going to die, from dementia or something else. We are born with a death sentence. There are literally hundreds of us around the world living beyond the diagnosis of

dementia. There is absolutely no reason to assume the pseudo death the sector currently supports.

Living beyond dementia is not possible.
All I have to say about that is what a load of bollocks! As mentioned in the last comment, there are hundreds, in fact more likely millions, of us living beyond the diagnosis of dementia. What we need is for the discourse of suffering and tragedy to stop, and for the myths to stop, and for the system to support us to live beyond the diagnosis of dementia. We all want to pass on the baton to others to start living beyond dementia, and for as long as possible, and to re-empower people with dementia to reclaim their pre-diagnosis lives.

Finally, having had many global conversations with others diagnosed with dementia about the terms 'living well with dementia', or 'living better with dementia', these terms are not palatable for everyone with dementia, whereas 'living beyond dementia' seems to be acceptable and far more palatable.

If those within the system don't know how to help people to live beyond dementia, all they need to do is ask one of us who is doing just that!

- The attitudes of researchers and health care professionals need to change on this.

- The language of dementia needs to change to better support living beyond dementia.

- Positive things are happening regarding living beyond dementia as many of us around the world are doing and speaking about publicly. It may not be possible for everyone, but it is possible for far more people than was once thought.

I firmly believe if we treat the symptoms of dementia as disAbilities, rather than a death sentence, as you would if you had a stroke or lost your legs in an accident, for example you would either get fitted with artificial limbs or a wheelchair, go through rehabilitation, and get on with your life accommodating the disAbilities, those of us living with dementia will live much better lives, and for longer, in spite of the diagnosis. The pseudo death role many currently take on will be replaced with living beyond dementia, using positive strategies and disAbility supports to manage the losses of function or capacity.

Myths are simply that. They are not fact, and we have to be very careful if deciding to believe in them that we are not simply supporting someone else's agenda, for example buying a product or supplement they are selling, or even signing up to a workshop that is being spruiked for the benefits of people with dementia, or any other false belief. If you don't stand up and speak for yourself, I can guarantee someone else will, and most simply do not know what you are feeling or experiencing, nor what is best for you.

——————————————

CHAPTER 15

Loneliness and Dementia

LONELINESS[1]

A sense of loneliness
So deep
It takes my breath away
Reminding me of those departed
Lingering inside my heart
Lost to the stigma of dementia
Tales of despair
Whisperings of days gone by
Deteriorating abilities
Sadness sitting just inside my soul
Yearning for my loss of self

(KATE SWAFFER 2014)

I'm not so sure the loneliness of dementia is any worse than when you are facing any other terminal disease or major crisis, except that the stigma and discrimination of dementia exacerbates the loneliness as so many cannot seem to get over their own fear of the disease and subsequently stop visiting us.

—————————————————————————

1   http://kateswaffer.com/2014/10/18/loneliness-2

There is a burden to dementia and any other illness that we must face alone. So much of how we feel is hard to put into words for others who are not on the same side of the fence to fully understand, one of the reasons support groups work so well. Some time ago we visited a friend who had just been diagnosed with lung cancer, and I could see the sadness behind his brave words and face, and the terrible burden he felt about the impact of his death on his wife and family. We had another friend facing this too, although much further down the track in this terrible disease. They have both since died.

There are so many things we feel we cannot say to each other, feelings and sadnesses that sit heavily inside our heart, causing at times an intense loneliness, and often isolating us from our loved ones. Our partner is desperate for us not to die or deteriorate, desperate for us to 'fight' the disease. Yet the person with the terminal disease eventually comes to terms with dying, accepting it as inevitable, what I call the 'we live until we die' philosophy. How do we tell the people we love we are okay with the prospect of dying, without it making them feel like we are giving up?

The loneliness really begins following a diagnosis of a terminal illness, as it is virtually impossible for one to think about anything other than their own impending losses... The person diagnosed has been given a death sentence, but their loved ones have also been given a death sentence – of their current existence – and a life looming in front of them without their loved one. On top of this, our culture has not taught us to talk openly about death and dying. As Norbert Elias once said, 'There is a tacit isolation of the... dying from the community of the living' (2001, p.2).

Through my blog, and other social media, I have made so many new friends, the depth of my sadness and the loss of old friendships, and the pure loneliness of dementia, has been seriously thwarted… And I am one of the lucky ones diagnosed with dementia, as many of my friends are still by my and our side, even though having people around me does not always take away the loneliness of dementia.

I often wrestle with a deep sense of loneliness. In my search for wisdom, I have re-read a Wakley Prize Essay, Dr Ishani Kar-Purkayastha's moving essay *An Epidemic of Loneliness* (2010); it was a timely reminder of the problems most recalcitrant to our research-based and outcome-driven health care providers.

Loneliness involves both social and emotional components – aloneness and sadness. It relates to the subjective difference between people's expectations of relationships and their social experience. It is a response to isolation of some kind, real or perhaps even imagined. I agree with Mother Teresa's quote about likening loneliness and feeling unwanted to a most terrible poverty.

But as is happening more often, I digress… Below I have quoted from Dr Kar-Purkayastha's essay:

> She lets out a forlorn noise that is neither laugh nor cry. 'Doctor', she asks, 'can you give me a cure for loneliness?' Her courage takes my breath away.
>
> I wish I could say yes. I wish I could prescribe her some antidepressants and be satisfied that I had done my best, but the truth is she's not clinically depressed. It's just that she has been left behind by a world that no longer revolves around her, not even the littlest bit of it.
>
> There are probably thousands like her. Men and women who have lived a lot and loved a lot. Men and women who are not yet done with being ferocious and bright but for whom time now stands empty as they wait in homes full of silence; their only misunderstanding to have lived to an age when they are no longer coveted by a society addicted to youth.

The depth and sense of my loneliness often takes my breath away, reminding me of the sadness of my loved ones who died in a nursing home, and of the desperate loneliness they must have felt in between our visits, and perhaps even during visits. The tales of sadness and loneliness many of my elderly friends tell are poignant, and often bring tears to my eyes. In my experience, older people who live with a partner have no idea and often show little understanding towards their peers living alone, facing old age and loneliness alone.

I am lucky enough to still have friends, but because of our ages, most of them are busy and working. Even having my husband give up work may not cure my loneliness, as it is bearing down on me as the symptoms of dementia take over more areas of my life. Having company does not always cure it. Often, not even joining a room full of my own friends would fill the gap; the reduced ability to fully and equally participate actually causes a deeper sense of loneliness. Just like dementia, there is no cure.

I don't write about loneliness to evoke or elicit pity or sympathy, but to help with understanding, for myself, and for others. I am often plagued by feeling of loneliness, that sometimes even stop me blogging. For me, social media and online support groups, and advocating for the human rights of people with dementia and older people, goes some way to filling the gap, but it does not fill it completely. Working for that six-month period last year helped to fill the gap and killed off some of the feelings of loneliness, and having colleagues again and a staff Christmas party to go to helped me a lot last Christmas. Not working, for younger people with a dementia, is not only a financial loss, but a loss of identity, of colleagues and of the many social gatherings, informal and formal, that fill one's soul.

However, most of my days, when I am at home, I am alone with my computer and cat, no visitors, few phone calls and my four walls.

No driver's licence, challenges catching public transport, the high cost of relying on taxis, changes to cognition and memory, deteriorating maths, writing and language skills, changes to interpersonal relationships, lost relationships, reduced problem-solving skills and many other changes due to dementia all go towards increasing the sense of loneliness.

It's not really possible to understand the added loneliness of living alone, even when I am home alone most days, as in the back of my mind, I know someone I love and who loves me is coming home later in the day. I cannot even begin to imagine what it would be like if I lived alone.

I've written many poems and blogs on loneliness and dementia, but no matter how often I write about it, I always feel there is so much more...

————————————————————————

CHAPTER 16

Prescribed Disengagement®

Dementia is the only disease or condition
The only terminal illness that I know of
Where patients are told to
Go home and give up
Rather than to fight for their lives

(KATE SWAFFER 2012)

Subsequent to my being diagnosed with younger onset frontotemporal dementia, probably semantic, in 2008, at the age of 49, health care professionals and service providers all told me the same thing: to give up work, give up study and go home and *live* for the time I had left. On the way, it was also suggested I put my end-of-life affairs in order – even though at no time was I told dementia is a terminal illness – and to get acquainted with aged care, including selecting a respite and residential care facility, sooner rather than later, so I could become used to it. My husband was told he would soon have to give up work to become a full-time family care partner.

Very quickly I termed this Prescribed Disengagement®, and thankfully I eventually chose to ignore it. Because

Prescribed Disengagement® is a term I came up with, I was advised to trademark it before someone else did, and hence have done so, and it has passed the very stringent criteria process and been listed in two categories:

> Class 41: Educational services relating to the diagnosis of dementia

> Class 44: Medical services relating to the diagnosis of dementia

It seems extraordinary that one day I was studying a tertiary degree, working full-time, volunteering, parenting two teenage boys and running a household, doing the shopping and gardening, living a very busy and full life with my husband and, the next day, told to give up life as I knew it and to *live* for the time left.

All of this advice was well-meaning, but it is based on a lack of education and preconceived expectations and myths about how people can or, as it seems is clear, misperceptions that we can't live beyond dementia, but only die from it. This sets people with dementia up to live a life without hope, without any sense of a future and destroys the notion of wellbeing

This Prescribed Disengagement® sets up a chain reaction of hopelessness and fear which negatively impacts a person's ability to be positive, resilient and proactive, ultimately affecting their wellbeing and quality of life. Without hope, it is a wonder anyone of us bother to make an effort to live at all.

After the diagnosis, when you are feeling like the darkest dark *will* put out the brightest candle, then being told to go home, get acquainted with aged care and get your end-of-life affairs in order, can only make you believe there is *no* hope. Taking away a person's hope, ultimately, and often very quickly, means they will simply give up.

I gave up paid employment aged 50 after my driver's licence was revoked; however, I should have been supported to continue to work. It is a legal duty not to discriminate against anyone with a disAbility and people with dementia have exactly the same legal rights to support with reasonable adjustments from an employer to remain employed as any other person, if they wish to be employed, for as long as possible.

Any person who has a disAbility, mental health or medical condition, including cognitive impairment, which impacts on their work, is eligible for services. The definition of disAbility is broad and is defined in the Disability Discrimination Act (1992) and does not exclude the disAbilities caused by the symptoms of dementia.

However, thanks to the support of the disAbility (with the emphasis on 'ability') services at the University of South Australia, I not only continued to study, completing two tertiary degrees post-diagnosis, I went on to complete a Master's of Science in Dementia Care at the University of Wollongong (2014). Continuing to study post-diagnosis meant I had to set up and use a lot of disAbility supports and strategies to be productive and ensure I lived a positive and meaningfully engaged life, with real purpose. It helped take away the focus from dementia and dying, to achievement. It also increased my neuroplasticity more than games on an iPad have the potential to do, and my resilience. Thankfully, at university, I was, and still am, viewed as a whole person, in the same way as any other disAbled person.

What's the cost?

The cost of this Prescribed Disengagement® sets up people with dementia to become *victims* or *sufferers*, their partners to eventually start behaving like martyrs, and to take over for the person diagnosed. It sets up people with dementia to believe there is no hope, there are no strategies to manage the symptoms of dementia, and more importantly, that it's not worthwhile trying to find any. It negatively impacts self-esteem, a person's finances, relationships and the ability to see any sort of positive future. Having dementia does not mean you have to give up living a pre-diagnosis life, nor living beyond dementia. For some, following a diagnosis of dementia, their whole life becomes about dementia and many seem to forget to keep living the other parts of their lives. This is another negative effect of the Prescribed Disengagement®.

Prescribed Disengagement® also takes away any power or control of the person diagnosed, giving it all to the family care partners and service providers. It is unhealthy, and wrong. Dementia is the only terminal illness I know of where people are told to go home and give up, rather than to fight for their lives.

Prescribing Disengagement® also lowers a person's own expectations about how they can live, and it lowers others' expectation about how we can function and live, including employers, health care professionals and service providers. For example, if I had experienced a stroke, I would have been authentically rehabilitated and supported to return to work, in whatever capacity possible. My employer would have been legally obliged to provide not only an alternative position for me if required, but to support any disAbilities. For people with younger onset dementia, this is extremely important and potentially could keep us living better lives for much longer, including continued employment.

It has the potential to completely disAble us emotionally, leading us to learned helplessness, as defined by Overmier:

> Learned helplessness arises from experiencing unpredictable and uncontrollable events – usually traumatic ones – and is reflected in reduced ability to cope with future life challenges; these challenges could be behavioural, psychological/ cognitive, or health related. The demonstrations that experiencing uncontrollable, unpredictable traumatic events leads to future failures to cope with environmental challenges are of considerable importance empirically and theoretically and they inform psychological treatment of depression and posttraumatic stress disorder and psychological science. (2013)

If when we are diagnosed we are told there is not hope, we are advised to give up work and our pre-diagnosis lives, and then counselled to prepare for end-of-life and aged care, it is highly possible that many people diagnosed with dementia take on a type of learned helplessness. Family members support it, not because they mean to disAble and disempower us, but because they are advised they will have to take over from us very soon, and so they do.

We need to break this negative and destructive cycle, and it has to start at the time of diagnosis and our immediate post-diagnostic support needs to reflect a more palatable and more ethical pathway of support.

Reclaiming my pre-diagnosis life

As we move towards creating and providing dementia-friendly communities, it links in with my belief that people with dementia must stay engaged in their pre-diagnosis lives, if they enjoy those things, for as long as possible and, for younger people, remain employed with assistance in the same way as any other disAbled person.

This will help to reduce the discrimination, stigma and isolation and will help others see that people with dementia are still very capable of contributing to their communities and society positively. As we have not been active in our own advocacy until recently, it is not yet the norm, and this affects how people treat us. It is a very recent phenomenon that people with dementia are included in the conversations that are about them. Sadly, staying engaged means many people with dementia are accused of lying about their diagnosis. Personally I prefer to ignore these doubters and continue to strive to live beyond dementia; it comes from the stigma still very present, and from ignorance. If I was doing well with cancer, no-one would doubt the diagnosis.

It is clear from the numbers of people with dementia who are standing up and speaking out as advocates that *there is still a good life to live even after a diagnosis of dementia.* We do not have to accept the Prescribed Disengagement® and give up our pre-diagnosis lives.

No, having dementia may not be as much fun as a birthday party, but there is no need to die that pseudo death upon diagnosis.

I recommend to everyone who has been diagnosed with dementia, and who has done what the dementia sector has prescribed, to ignore this well-meaning but unconstructive advice and *re-invest in life.*

We must reclaim our pre-diagnosis life.

I'm not talking about money, but about living beyond dementia and continuing to live the same life as your pre-diagnosis one for as long as possible. Sure, get your wills and other end-of-life issues sorted out because dementia is a terminal illness and one where you will most likely lose legal capacity, but there is no need not to work hard to slow down the deterioration, nor to stop doing the things you have always done, if you still want to do them.

Models of care

The medical model of Prescribed Disengagement® versus the disAbility or social pathway of support and authentic rehabilitation and remaining engaged in pre-diagnosis lives is worth outlining. Whilst they are not specifically modelled on evidence-based practice, the models on the following pages, based on my own experience, outline plainly the differences, although there is emerging evidence to support this pathway.

Prescribed Disengagement®

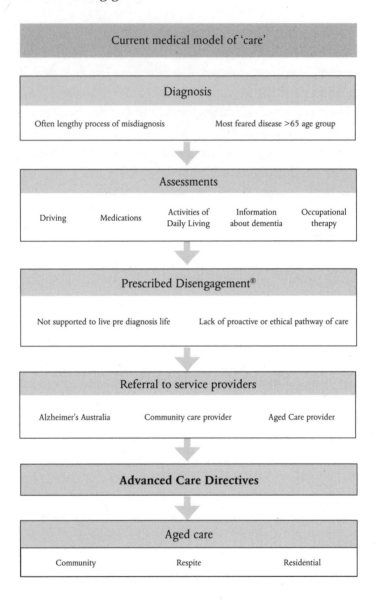

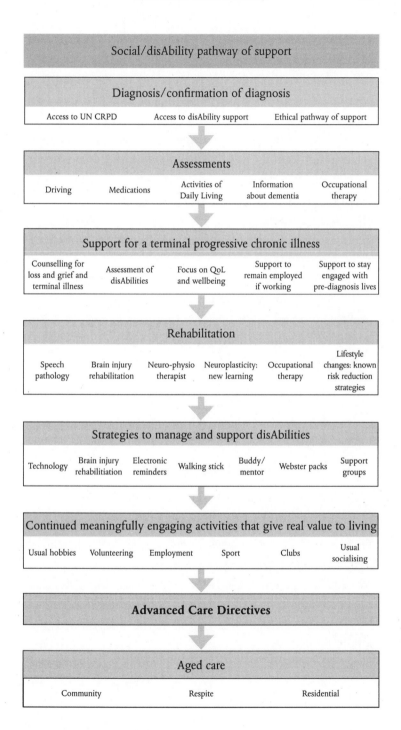

Prescribed Disengagement® supports and exacerbates ignorance, social inequality, exclusion, stigma, isolation, fear and discrimination, and dementia is the only disease I have heard of where you are told to *give up* rather than *fight for your life*.

This is, simply put, a preposterous and negative prescription. It is also unethical and immoral. Unfortunately drug companies support it, as medicating for behaviours is good for their bottom line. Recommending holistic or other interventions that do not involve prescriptions of pharmacology is not on their agenda, nor, sadly, that of many researchers.

It is important to focus on living, and quality of life and wellbeing, or perceived wellbeing, as for too long this has been ignored. Consider prescribing or asking for these, instead of Prescribed Disengagement®:

- Positive psychosocial interventions.

- Non-pharmacological interventions.

- DisAbility/social model of support, not medical model.

- Provide authentic brain injury rehabilitation.

- Support pre-diagnosis life, including employment if person has younger onset dementia.

Imagine if the medical community told people with cancer to get their end-of-life affairs in order and go home and live for the time they had left, or perhaps even decided not to tell them they had cancer because it is a difficult diagnosis for them to deal with.

When diagnosed with dementia, I was offered the following pathway:

- *Referral to service provider to provide support at home, respite or residential aged care,* Alzheimer's Association or an aged care provider (I was too young to qualify for aged care).

- Link or key worker – at the time, funding was unavailable for this service.

- Memory Loss course and support group.

- Activities, e.g. bingo, art, coffee groups, art therapy, hair brushing, smelling fresh flowers or pot pourri, stroking an animal, a visit to a herb farm or a flower show.

- Safe Return bracelet.

- Planning for the future, getting my end-of-life affairs in order (I still believe this needs to be done).

- Coping with 'behaviour' changes.

- Preparing my home.

- Community and respite aged care – advised to start soon, so I would get used to it.

- Residential care.

- No referral to disAbility or employment adviser, which leads to:

  » increased stigma, discrimination, isolation, loneliness and social inequality

  » higher risk of depression and apathy

  » negative impact on progression of dementia and a very negative impact on my ability to be positive, or to 'fight for my life'.

The University of South Australia disAbility support services, on the other hand, offered me this pathway:

- *Referral to Disability Adviser to provide support to continue with studies.*

- Mentor and buddy.

- Disability Access Plan (diagnosis accepted with medical confirmation letter from my neurologist).

- Alternative assessments and exams.

- Counselling for loss and grief.

- Note taker and/or podcasts.

- Strategies for students, e.g.:

  » planning for completion of degree

  » time management

  » managing reading and writing

  » study skills, library assistance, etc.

- Supportive aids, as required.

- Disability equipment and Assisted Technology.

- Referral to careers and employment, or referral to disAbility career sector on how to stay in employment if still employed, or to gain employment, which led to:

  » reduced stigma, discrimination, isolation and loneliness

  » minimal loss of equality

  » meaningful positive engagement, sense of valued achievement and chance of decreased progression of dementia, apathy and depression.

There is no comparison, and the fact I have completed three university degrees, post-diagnosis, speaks for itself.

Friday, 18th April, 2014

RE: Ms Kate Swaffer

To Whom It May Concern,

I am the treating neurologist of the above named patient.

I have treated her for a number of years for semantic dementia. A semantic dementia is a focal neurodegenerative process where the patient has difficulty understanding the meaning of words.

The severity of the condition has progressed with time. She is quite disabled and has word finding difficulty. She is currently suffering from short-term memory loss, word finding difficulty and dyslexia.

She does have a number of other neurological and spinal issues which also impact on her health including a chronic neck condition and severe pain of the lower back and limbs.

There is no known treatment for the neurodegenerative process and the spinal issues are being treated with medication.

Clearly these conditions would have a significant impact on her academic performance.

She has a number of neuropsychological reports which have documented the severity of the condition.

In terms of the neurodegenerative process she would require more time for study and during her exams. The pain and spinal issues would also negatively impact on her condition and comfort levels. She clearly would require consideration of being given more time to complete her studies and during exams. She does have quite a severe physical impairment with respect to the spinal issues and frequently is unable to sit for any length of time during my consultations with her.

I fully support her registering with the disability service and I hope this letter is helpful in providing possible strategies that can be recommended.

Copied verbatim from a medical confirmation
letter provided by my neurologist

It is time all people with dementia and their families stood up for better advice and services that enhance our quality of life and wellbeing, and that support for 'fighting for our lives' is offered, as it is for every other disease and terminal illness. Misguided and preconceived misconceptions about the symptoms of dementia are still being used to support telling us to give up living our pre-diagnosis lives.

The recognition of the symptoms as disAbilities would assist with a more equitable and dementia-friendly experience for the person with dementia after diagnosis. In contrast to the medical model, the disAbility patway of support is positive and supports continued engagement with our pre-diagnosis lives. One of the definitions of a myth is 'an unproved or false collective belief that is used to justify a social institution' (Dictionary.com). I believe it is this myth that many in the health care and aged care sectors continue to support to justify their lack of dignified person-centred care.

In the next chapter, I will go into more detail about the disAbility model, or options offered to me by the Disability Adviser at the University of South Australia, explaining the contrast and how helpful it was.

In the meantime, I am beyond thrilled to report that I am part of a research team currently applying for funding to conduct research into moving away from this Prescribed Disengagement® we receive at diagnosis, to the prescription of engagement, looking at the value and implications for a much better quality of life, and, who knows, the slowing down of the progression of the disease. Not long ago, I felt like I had been banging my head against a solid brick wall about this, but now there seems to be a small group of academics and clinicians who want to investigate it further, and, importantly for me, who are including me in the process.

In February 2015, I ran a pre-conference workshop called *Diagnosed with Dementia: What next?* at the National Dementia Congress in Melbourne, where I also gave a keynote presentation, *Young Onset Dementia: Reclaiming my life today*. A friend living with dementia, Maxine Thomson, ran it with me, as we co-developed it.

The workshop was with a small group of people working in the dementia sector: nurses, psychologists, social workers and so on, all keen to provide better support to people with younger onset dementia. The workshop included them working in small groups on the pathway of support they either provide, or that was currently available to people with younger onset dementia, and then to do the same for a person who had a recoverable stroke.

The most interesting part of this, for me, was that in my preparation I printed off a number of relevant, but also very basic, help sheets to assist them with care plans for someone with dementia, including younger onset dementia. I then went to the Stroke Foundation, and printed off the National Stroke management guidelines, all 167 pages of them!

The care plans they came up with for the person with younger onset dementia included:

- Diagnosis

- Information to client and family

- Talking/asking about feelings/needs/family needs

- Empower/engage/individualised services/PCC

- Identify changes, goals, barriers

- ACDs (Advanced Care Directives)

- Referral to respite/care/link workers
- If possible, support to stay at work
- Support groups
- Information, e.g. managing money, symptom 'management'

The care plan for the person who had a stroke included:

- Diagnosis
- Assessment
- Information to client and family
- Rehabilitation
  - » Occupational Therapy
  - » Physiotherapy
  - » Speech Pathology
  - » Walking/mobility rehab
  - » Dietician
  - » Psychologist
  - » Social worker
  - » Specialised fine motor skill rehab
  - » Counselling, including for grief and loss
  - » Support groups

The second very interesting part of this workshop was that, in reality, the first case study was quite challenging for many in the group, due to the fact that there are very few services for people with young onset dementia (or dementia generally), and because the post-diagnostic support offered by the sector is very limited, and misses for the most part, beyond end of life, managing symptoms, and aged care services, any real interventions. The contrast was quite stark, as the ease with which the second case study was tackled, and care plans evolved, was quick, and easily followed national guidelines. ￣

Australia will soon release their first national clinical guidelines for dementia, and although I feel they lack enough proactive post diagnostic support for us, they are at least a good start.

The value of disAbility and social support

At the University of South Australia, I was referred by my lecturers to the DisAbility Adviser and set up with an Access Plan, active for the continuation and completion of my studies. This Access Plan evolved as the symptoms demanded, changing in the same way it would if I had an acquired brain injury, or a disease like multiple sclerosis where symptoms are regularly changing. I was treated as a whole person, with support for the disAbilities, rather than advised to disengage and give up. Following graduation in Bachelor of Arts and then a Bachelor of Psychology, both post-diagnosis, it demonstrated that treating the symptoms of dementia as disAbilities to be dealt with and supported, rather than managing them in ways that restricted and hindered me, were vital to my general wellbeing, my motivation, and not only my sense of meaningful engagement, but real achievement, giving me a sense of real value in the world.

The other significant value of study is it is a method of neuroplasticity and brain training. If I had been referred to a brain injury unit, I would have been proactively *supported* to live the best life possible with whatever *injury or disease*

I have. Suggesting disengaging from my meaningful life and taking up activities others think might sustain my brain and soul is irrational and offensive. The disAbility sector sees everyone as whole human beings and helps with strategies so the person can continue functioning as well as possible in their own way. The significant and positive impact of being meaningfully and positively engaged is paramount to a person's wellbeing, their ability to be resilient and positive, their motivation to fight against the symptoms of dementia, and their ability to better manage the emotional toll of the diagnosis. Dr Norman Doidge's two books, *The Brain that Changes Itself* and *The Brain's Way of Healing*, fully describe with anecdotal evidence in his first book, then with evidence based research in the second book, how important neuroplasticity is, and its relevance to people with a dementia.

Serious about living beyond dementia

Alzheimer's Disease International has the following charter:

> I can live well with dementia.[1]

For some time, I had thought that phrase was positive and helpful. However, not only does no-one tell us how to 'live well with dementia', they don't even tell us that living well with, or living beyond, dementia is possible. Many people with dementia also find this term unrealistic and therefore perhaps unachievable.

Public and health care professionals' perceptions of people with dementia, fuelled by the negative discourse used in the media and by most people when they are writing or talking about people with dementia, continue to suggest it

---

1   www.alz.co.uk/global-dementia-charter

is simply not possible to live well with dementia, or indeed beyond the diagnosis.

A colleague and dear friend of mine, Dr Shibley Rahman, wrote some time ago on this topic as part of a Facebook discussion with some care partners, many of whom mostly insist we are all 'suffering'.

> *The concept of living well with dementia is not an attempt to sanitise people's experiences of dementia, nor to be a way by which some feel guilty or uncomfortable that perhaps they are not doing enough themselves to be able to live well with dementia. It is a concept that is meant to convey that there could be more constructive ways of promoting well-being and better quality of life for people with a diagnosis of dementia.*

Living beyond dementia is now my preferred term to support anyone who has been diagnosed with a dementia, as a way of helping them to think about the possibility of living more positively with dementia than is currently thought possible, prescribed or taught. Fingers crossed! I hope it is more helpful, and feedback so far has been really encouraging. The terms living well or living better too easily imply that someone may not be living well, may not be 'doing enough' to be able to live well, or the term living better (or worse) too easily compares us to someone else's version of what that is.

It could easily be seen as being too prescriptive, and as either ignoring or dishonouring the very real challenges of being diagnosed with dementia, which is a terminal, progressive, chronic illness that ultimately 'steals' our functioning and capacity until we die. For some time now, there has been a global conversation around the terms living well and living better with dementia, but perhaps these are not very helpful terms.

Since being diagnosed with dementia, I have learned to *live beyond the diagnosis of dementia.*

It did not happen easily, or straight away, and for the first 18 months or so, I was spiraling downhill rapidly, with no thoughts of it ever being possible to live beyond dementia, or to continue to excel and exceed my expectations, or to continue to reach any of my goals.

Once I discovered I could view, and more importantly manage, the symptoms as disAbilities, and found strategies to support them to allow me to function, albeit differently to when I did not have dementia, I started to see another way.

As I developed my thinking on dementia through the lens of my own lived experience, including coming up with the phrase Prescribed Disengagement®, I started to think about ways to combat this negative prescription of giving up our pre-diagnosis lives.

As a result of this, my ability to live more positively and productively with dementia increased. Yes, I know this will change one day, and as some well-meaning nurse told me one day after a presentation I had given about non pharmacological interventions for dementia, 'It will get you in the end'…but that does not matter, as I was born with a death sentence anyway, just as she was!

Being diagnosed with dementia was certainly not a reason to die straight away or give up on striving to live positively and beyond the symptoms dementia. I was not at the end stage of the disease, and therefore to suggest I give up my pre-diagnosis life was extremely unhelpful, and I'd go as far as saying it is also completely unethical, as is the fact that many doctors make a decision not to inform their patients they have dementia…as if that is okay!

Living beyond dementia is, I believe, what we need to learn to do, and what health care professionals need to support us to do. On top of that, if we can get rid of Prescribed Disengagement®, and have health care providers offer us proactive, rehabilitative and enabling post-diagnostic pathways of support, with strategies and support for the disAbilities that the symptoms of dementia insist on giving us, many more people with dementia will live much better lives beyond the diagnosis, and the current pathway of loss, despair and a focus on our deficits will be reduced. It will also keep us living in our own homes and communities much longer, and I do believe that research will eventually prove this. I have faith in this, although like Stephen Hawking had to do when he disproved his own theory, I also accept I may be wrong.

I stopped crying a few weeks after being diagnosed, and ultimately took action to actively ditch the PLOM (Poor Little Old Me) disease that I had for a long time after the diagnosis, and to get back on with living.

We are all born with a death sentence, but do we wake up every day focused on that without bothering to strive to live as well as possible? I know of no-one who wakes up every day waiting to die.

When diagnosed with any other terminal illness, most people strive to live as well as possible with it, and to fight it, and importantly the medical community proactively supports them with every medical or holistic step and support to do so.

So why, when we are diagnosed with dementia, would we want to give up striving to live beyond dementia upon diagnosis?

Personally, even though a diagnosis of dementia is not as much fun as a birthday party, I do think it is far preferable to accept that a diagnosis of dementia does not have to mean the instant death of the life we had before the diagnosis. I believe it is very important to keep challenging perceptions of dementia, as without doing that, nothing will ever change.

One must ponder, is it easier to live well or beyond a diagnosis of any illness, including dementia, without adequate funds? The following is a comment posted privately to me on Facebook about a post on my new blog, *Living Beyond Dementia*, titled 'Living well, living better, or living beyond dementia?'

> *Thank you!! I have heard so many negative comments about the whole 'living well with dementia' campaign. Maybe some people have money to do the things they did and are not restricted by their symptoms – I am not one of them. I think people need to hear the good and the bad. This life is NOT easy, but it's NOT the stigma people think. There is, however, a balance. I love the phrase Living Beyond much better!*

This was my reply:

> *I love the term too as it does not subtly negate the less pleasant sides of dementia and I agree living well is too hard for too many to accept, and reasonably so too. I've also thought a lot about the difference having money can make to what's possible and know far more people with dementia are living with very limited funds, which adds to the negative impact of the diagnosis.*

This conversation brings me to talk about the impact of dementia and what many people tell me they experience after a diagnosis, which is that they end up being almost on the poverty line after the diagnosis, and that this impacts on their ability to live well, in any sense of that word, or beyond the diagnosis.

Perhaps though, with a change in the system and our post-diagnostic support, and moving away from Prescribed Disengagement®, it may not impact our ability to live beyond the diagnosis as much as it does currently.

I am not by any stretch of the imagination a capitalist, and in fact my husband says that if he won the lottery (he buys the occasional ticket; I don't as I dislike gambling), he probably would not tell me if he'd won, as I'd be likely to give half of it away to a homeless organisation, The Big Issue SA, and the other half to Dementia Alliance International! But having money allows one to have freedom, and more importantly in the case of a terminal, progressive, chronic illness like dementia, to bring in services and support, and to be able to engage in a lifestyle and activities including travel and leisure that definitely increase one's perceived wellbeing and quality of life. In reality, most countries' health care systems barely provide proper health care, let alone anything else!

So my two questions on the topic are: *Is living beyond dementia, or in fact, beyond any other terminal of chronic condition or disease, as simple as having available spare cash? Is it possible to live well without money?*

To be really honest, I am not sure if money is the only important thing in the scenario, as I most definitely do believe our *attitude has a lot to do with it*, but without money, ultimately, I suspect it is really tough to live well beyond any health issue or crisis, no matter what one's definition of living well is.

For example, I have two friends who actually choose to be homeless, who say they prefer to live in the parklands, and away from the 'trappings of money'. They find life is far less complicated, and it is their choice.

I also know people who talk about their own lives as if their financial resources have nothing to do with their lifestyle, and yet, for example, to become an artist or a writer or an actor, without financial resources coming from somewhere or from someone else, it is so much easier when you are financially supported while you are struggling to make any money from your art. Without this support, it would be almost impossible to live or to bring up a family.

Without my husband still working, life might be quite different for us. Although, having both grown up in low income families, we have been very careful with our money and saved for tough times. That has helped as well.

Being poor is hard work at the best of times; I know as I have been very poor a few times in my life. But add in a terminal illness, and that most definitely may mean any sense of living well, or beyond, the disease is almost impossible.

The members of Dementia Alliance International are serious about empowering and teaching other people with dementia to remain engaged and to find strategies to support living beyond the diagnosis of dementia, and that it is possible for some of us with their appropriate and proactive support.

The Scottish Dementia Working Group is serious about living beyond dementia, as are the members of the European, Australian, Irish, Japanese and Ontario Dementia Working Groups. People with dementia make up the membership in all of these groups, and we are living proof people can live beyond the diagnosis of dementia, and can and do contribute significantly and positively to society.

Sooner or later, there will be enough anecdotal evidence, by the sheer numbers of us doing this, for others to believe it possible, and more importantly, to promote it. People with dementia are all working together to support the voices of each other, and ourselves to improve our own lives and futures. As our collective voices become louder, the health and dementia care sectors, and even those family care partners who insist on our experiences being only of 'suffering', will eventually see there is another way. I am deadly serious about living beyond the diagnosis of dementia, and being as proactive as is humanly possible. After all, the alternative is less than inviting.

CHAPTER 17

Dementia as a DisAbility

DISABLED

I am able
To perform activities
Willing to operate
At my own level
I may be challenged
But I am capable
And operating
Not inoperative
I can function
And I am only restricted
By those around me
Who choose to dis me
Yes I am able
Capable and talented
Equipped to live
A worthwhile life

(KATE SWAFFER 2015)

Treating symptoms in the early stages of dementia, as the gateway to supporting disAbilities, not managing them in ways that restrict and hinder, and managing emotional changes with counselling and positive engagement, rather than treating the symptoms with drugs, have become paramount to my wellbeing and perceived longevity.

However, negative attitudes about not only dementia but also disAbility are alive and well, and the battle to overcome these continues for us all.

A few years ago, and with some apprehension alongside a strong sense of interest, I attended Pathways 9 conference, which I remain grateful was made possible due to the provision of a grant for my attendance. After applying and being selected to represent the '*disAbled*' student body of the University of South Australia, I felt not only a sense of achievement, but a strong sense of responsibility to properly stand up for these students. In cahoots with the other grant beneficiary (Julie), it was moderately amusing to think that the recipients of this grant were two students, one who could not see where she is going, and the other (me), who often cannot remember where she is going, nor where she has been...a likely pair!

As my own disAbility is not easily 'visible', I often feel like a fraud amongst those visibly disAbled, and the overwhelming feeling I came away with from this conference is that I disliked the label of *disAbility*, and the many negative connotations that word implies. Upon discussion with several others, it seems to be a strong feeling amongst many of us who have not been born *disAbled*, or who have not been diagnosed at an early age.

I did then, and in some ways still do, find the words *disAbility* and *disAbled* patronising and humiliating, in the same way I prefer not to be referred to as *demented* and even more so as my disease progresses because it undermines who I am, and in some way makes me feel incomplete as a person. However, in the context of care and post-diagnostic support, having the symptoms treated and managed as disAbilities is far more positive and helpful.

It was highly confronting arriving at the registration desk and reception for a conference for university staff and disAbled students, as I had not come to terms with the fact I have many 'disAbilities'. My response to this experience was to question the term disAbility, and whether it disAbled me more. The words 'disAbility' and 'disAbled', in relation to my progression of illness and its disAbling impact on my life, feel like they define me as a person but are far preferable to being called demented. Of course, I would prefer you just to call me Kate, a person with some different needs to others and diverse ways of operating in this world, not someone with dementia or a disAbility. It is probably why I started writing with a capital A in disAbility.

At this conference, I listened to an academic, Kevin Murfatt, a man who is legally blind, a lecturer at Deakin University, and at the time he was head of Vision Australia. He suggested 'Employment is how we define ourselves'. I would suggest education is one of the main keys to employment, which highlights the need for equity to enable individuals to 'define themselves'. Equal status is the most important thing to 'disAbled' peoples, higher than anything else including getting to know people, including for people with dementia.

Despite equal opportunity and anti-discrimination legislation, technological advances, and a growing awareness of rights to full social inclusion for people who have a disAbility, in the 22 years since the enactment of the Disability Discrimination Act (1992), employment of people who have a disAbility in Australia has declined, while for other Australians employment levels have increased.

Kevin discussed an instrument[1] he validated in his PhD that can uncover those deep and almost instinctual negative attitudes of even 'true believers', one that he himself has used approximately 12 times, and still shows him to have negative attitudes towards some groups in the community.

Examples of discrimination were considered such as the first female lead trumpet player in Germany, who not only had to fight to keep her winning position because she was female, but it took 15 years to receive pay equal to a male. In this case, and for the first time in history, the auditions were done behind a screen from the judges, and only because the son of one of the judges was auditioning. Women are still struggling with things such as equal pay, and still have a long way to go in many areas.

He also outlined the path to real attitude change and social inclusion for people who have a disAbility. His thesis 'Attitude change in employment of people who have a disAbility' is set in Ecological Systems Theory and found that direct experience with people who have a disAbility, rather than constructed scenarios, is the key to positive attitude change and that future research should utilise the powerful role stereotyped groups themselves have in attitude change through their own development and interaction with the environment.

It's a very interesting read. He also commented that he believed student evaluations of lecturers and courses were not only worthwhile, but assisted with the management of discrimination in positive ways, and in this way, having people with dementia start to evaluate and audit services may also go some way to actually bringing about real change. This is extremely relevant in the dementia-friendly communities initiatives and campaigns around the world, as

1   Questionnaire available via www.implicit.harvard.edu.

without people with dementia evaluating what is and what is not dementia-friendly it is not fully possible for people without dementia to know.

Most people understand racism, for example, as an attitude or set of attitudes towards individuals or groups, and prejudice to be the act of discrimination. While this may be an easy way of clarifying the terms, closer examination highlights different aspects of racism, and therefore of discrimination. The focus on racism being grounded in prejudicial, irrational and fanatical beliefs tends to focus our attention on the beliefs and actions of individuals. However, if we view discrimination as social and cultural rather than individual, our focus leads us to the way discrimination works behind our backs. Discrimination against those living with illness is often unseen. As a group or community we can participate in racist practices or actions without necessarily holding racist beliefs. This form of racism focuses on discrimination and is often described by the term 'institutional racism', which highlights the systemic processes that reproduce disadvantage. However, while institutional racism draws our attention to the workings of the state and other institutions and therefore their actions, we should continue to recognise individual racism and the role of beliefs, which transfer into the actions of discrimination. We often think with our beliefs but very rarely think about them, which works against those of us with disAbility and illness.

If the symptoms of dementia were treated as disAbilities, the negative impact on the person, their family, and society would be far less. We would be given assistance to remain employed or to live beyond dementia, which in turn would increase our social inclusion and social equality. This would decrease the isolation, stigma, and discrimination and would also reduce the negative economic impact on the person, their family and society.

We should be given strategies to assist us to live with the unique challenges of dementia: counselling to remain engaged with our pre-diagnosis activities, a dis*Ability* plan, assisted technologies, dis*Ability* equipment, mentoring, and even note takers or memory loss reading logs to help us function fully. This would ensure we are treated with dignity and as whole and individual human beings. At the ADI conference in Taipei in 2013, these things were recommended as slowing the progression of dementia, even though the year before when I presented them at the ADI conference in London, I was almost laughed off the stage:

- Positive psychosocial interventions

- Non-pharmacological interventions

- Neuroplasticity training

- Exercise and cognitive fitness

- Authentic brain injury rehabilitation

- Focus on wellbeing and QoL (quality of life)

In my first volume of poetry I wrote a poem called 'disAbled', also at the beginning of this chapter. A lady I met at ADI in London in 2012 living with dementia asked if she could read it out to a group she meets with in her area.

This is what she wrote back to me:

> I was speaking at a stakeholders conference in xxxxxx this week and read your poem again and it went down so well I told them about who you were and they took the message on board. ... I went to a 'talking heads' group where folk living with dementia were meant to be sharing strategies for coping (not care partners). I was the only one in the group living by

myself and when I was describing my systems (which break down of course now and again and have to be revamped) no-one else seemed to be interested in having any they just said oh X does that (spouse/care partner), it made me sad as I feel it disAbles them.

The way doctors and service providers dish out Prescribed Disengagement® has to be part of the reason people diagnosed with dementia give up even bothering to try and live beyond dementia. This prescription takes away all hope of a future, and fills us with fear and foreboding.

I have no idea how we can encourage people with dementia to even engage in the idea they can take action to enable their own lives, by ways of healthy lifestyle, neuroplasticity exercises, and so on, but I feel it is important we keep trying to.

These things do make a difference, they may not cure us, but they may slow down the rate at which dementia progresses for many people and they definitely increase the sense of wellbeing. There is a body of research growing to support this now, and yet people with dementia are not being told by their health professionals to engage in these things. Holistic, positive psychosocial and non-pharmacological interventions are a very real part of helping ourselves with any disease, and a few Western doctors are even starting to believe in them.

The latest research on risk reduction for dementia includes reducing isolation, choosing healthier lifestyle factors, including reducing or better managing blood pressure, cholesterol, diabetes and obesity, as well as neuroplasticity through new learning. Common sense would suggest to me that these things will also work to slow down the progression of the disease, and there is emerging evidence this may well be so.

If you were diagnosed with cancer, I feel sure you would engage in all sorts of healthy interventions, not just the medical options, so why not with dementia? It is curious to me that this particular diagnosis seems to make people only focus on the diagnosis, and re-diagnosis, and then the re-diagnosis, and re-diagnosis, and not on how to overcome the symptoms of the disease in more positive ways. I guess this is a search for new treatment options, but perhaps to the detriment of living a more positive life.

Of course, we all run our own race, which is exactly as it should be, but we do need to question, is the race so many people with dementia are running largely due to the Prescribed Disengagement®? Personally, I think it is.

About two years ago I met with an art therapist who is doing amazing things here with art and other therapy, and she is proving beyond doubt that positive meaningful engagement makes a difference. She told me stories of people with dementia who had not been able to stay focused for more than a few minutes, and, after being involved in the therapy she had set up, who could focus, uninterrupted, for two hours. Of course, there is limited evidence to support this, but she and the loving family and friends also see it happening. To me, it is simply more proof that it is worth engaging us to remain involved and active with our pre-dementia lives. Art does not do it for me, but writing and listening to music does. We all have our own unique likes and dislikes. Music is another intervention or recreation shown to improve mood, memories and language, and it would be worthwhile seeing the documentary 'Alive Inside' if you can, or at least looking up the clips on YouTube. The late Oliver Sacks did research into the effects of music, and the footage of Henry, and how he comes alive inside, is remarkable.

I believe there is a sense of what Martin Luther King described as 'the degenerating sense of "nobodiness"' (1963) amongst many disAbled people, especially those who are struggling with mental, terminal or chronic illness, old age and dementia. It is therefore imperative we aspire to change views about disAbility and, in my view, even the terms applied to us, and to fight for complete dignity and equality through transformation of services and attitudes.

There is often a feeling of disconnection as we struggle with the notion of a level playing field, as well as the feeling of 'otherness' as we reach out for services that are labelled in ways that make us feel even more different to others, and therefore marginalise us. We must continue to battle against the stereotypes, to break with the traditions that are steeped in bias, stigma and discrimination that maintain the lack of equity for the sick and disAbled, and that isolate us.

Dementia can too easily represent the end of dreaming, a long and unforgiving one-way odyssey into obscurity, clouded in a thick and unforgiving fog.

As I said at the beginning of this chapter, if we treat the symptoms of dementia as disAbilities, rather than a death sentence, as you would if you lost your legs in an accident – you would either get fitted with artificial limbs or a wheelchair, or go through rehabilitation – many more of us would simply get on with our lives accommodating our particular disAbilities, for as long as possible.

Stigma and Dementia

The stigma and ignorance continue
Systemic
Endemic
Passively working against us

Our human rights quietly denied
Fuelled by the exclusion of people with dementia
In all areas of life
On Boards and in research

Well-meaning people without dementia
Making decisions for us
Presenting about us
Whilst all this well-meaning talk takes place

It continues to be 'about us without us'
As very few are yet
Walking the talk
Of their own hypothetical advocacy

Whilst this keeps happening
Isolation
Discrimination, and
The stigma lives on

(KATE SWAFFER 2015)

The definition of stigma and the role it plays in defining the experience of people with dementia is well documented. Erving Goffman (1963) refers to stigma as 'spoiled identity'; Link and Phelan (2001) discuss it in terms of persons being negatively labelled, a loss of status and power, discrimination and stereotyping. Stigma affects a number of things when considering dementia, including the person's willingness to seek diagnosis, to seek support once diagnosed, and a lack of willingness to participate in research (Burgener and Berger 2008; Garand *et al.* 2009; Milne 2010). The care provided is also of a lower standard due to stigma within the health care profession, and services are distorted (Benbow and Jolley 2012; Devlin, MacAskill and Stead 2007; Milne 2010). Stigma increases the feelings of shame (Scheff 1990), and more recently ADI (2012) also reported people with dementia still feel a deep sense of shame. The Alzheimer's Society of Ireland (2008) reported on two types of stigma, one as external, that is stigma towards the person, and the other as internal stigma, where the person feels shame about themselves, or that they are 'less of a person' because of the symptoms of dementia. For timely diagnosis, more appropriate care, and to improve the quality of life for people with dementia, it is essential we reduce the stigma.

Stigma affects more than just wellbeing and quality of life for people with dementia and their families. Language, inclusion and providing dementia-friendly communities are important in the reduction of stigma, and without positive change, stigma will continue to be a significant burden on people with dementia. Stigma is still a salient feature of the experience of people with dementia (Batsch, Mittelman and ADI 2012; Ryan 2006; Hodkinson 2011; Mackenzie 2006), and because of this I have explored the existence of stigma within the dementia literature. It is apparent there is a lack of research focused on the effect or feeling of stigma specifically from the perspective of the person with dementia, and how stigma might be exacerbated by the use of incorrect information and inappropriate language used to describe people with dementia (Garand *et al.* 2009; Vincent, in DPS News 2014). The Honourable Kelly Vincent, MLC, leader of Dignity4Disability in South Australia, says, when communicating with people with disAbilities, that they are the experts; so too are those people diagnosed with dementia.

I have explored stigma in the literature, looking at it in a new way by questioning whether the researchers exacerbate stigma, even though their intent is to promote positive change. Considering the lack of inclusion of people with dementia in the cohorts being studied, it is still very much 'about people with dementia, without them', which cannot give a true picture of the issues at hand for this group, also serving to reinforce the stigma. Caregiver stigma has been explored often (Dean 2011a; Mackenzie 2006; Phillipson *et al.* 2012; Werner *et al.* 2012) but there is very little on the stigma as experienced directly by people with dementia. No longer can this expertise be ignored as people with dementia are the experts through the lived experience, and not including them in research not only stigmatises them, but it hinders the validity of the research. This is important as much of the published research is biased through the use of family care partners as the main cohort group, or having them in attendance when people with dementia are interviewed, and so the care partner voice remains the main voice in the dementia and stigma research.

There is a significant body of evidence to draw upon when reviewing stigma and language, and the literature appears to show more positive attitudes. However, this may be a socially acceptable veneer covering up the embedded and unconscious negative attitudes that drive human behaviour, expressed as stigma and discrimination.

It is therefore imperative we aspire to change views of and about people with dementia, and begin to include them in the research and conversations about them. Ken Clasper (2014) writes a blog about living with dementia, and said, '…we wish to raise awareness of dementia, is that we all live on hope, that we can in our own little way go a long way to remove the stigma which we hear of every day in dementia'. People with dementia are raising their voices all around the world, as they want to be part of the conversations and research, and until they are included, the stigma will continue. Evidence of this are groups like the Scottish Dementia Working Group (established in 2002), the European Dementia Working Group (2012), and the Australian Dementia Advisory Committee (2013), the first groups globally for people with dementia where membership is exclusive to them, and they are supported by their respective Alzheimer's Societies. They all advocate for a review of the language being used about them, for inclusion, reducing stigma, increasing education and awareness as the way forward in reducing stigma, and this activism is starting to be noticed (Bartlett 2014).

In the *World Alzheimer's Report 2012: Overcoming the Stigma of Dementia* (Batsch *et al.* 2012, p.23) out of 2068 UK respondents to their survey, 83 per cent were care partners and only 6 per cent were people living with a diagnosis of dementia, and in Spain there were only 3 per cent people with dementia versus 77 per cent care partners. The voice of others about and over people with dementia continues, and if the peak international body advocating for people with dementia is not able to access a better cohort of people with dementia, it not only highlights the challenges for researchers, it continues to stigmatise people with dementia through exclusion. Of course, there are challenging ethical and methodological considerations with working with people with dementia, with other issues such as capacity to give consent, which may also change during the course of the research, their vulnerability, and the possible emotional toll of participating in research (Pesonen, Remes and Isola 2011). It is no longer acceptable to do research about children, the disAbled or the LGBTI community, without them, so I wonder why it is still being done without people with dementia. This report cannot claim to have reported accurately on the stigma felt by people with dementia.

It is my belief we will not significantly reduce the stigma people with dementia feel, which leads to discrimination, exclusion and isolation, without first including them, and then changing the way we talk about or refer to them.

In 2012, a report on stigma in Australia exposed how the general community view dementia in general, and especially people diagnosed with dementia. Its findings found that 50.8 per cent of the respondents agreed that people with dementia cannot be expected to have a meaningful conversation, and 11.7 per cent of respondents said they would avoid spending much time with a person who had dementia. I know that was three years ago, but I feel we still have such a long way to go!

'Exploring Dementia and Stigma Beliefs' which describes the results of a pilot study which asked 616 Australians for their views about people with dementia. The study was conducted by Dr Lyn Phillipson and colleagues at the Centre for Health Initiative at the University of Wollongong.

Additionally, a percentage of respondents agreed that people with dementia:

- can be irritating – 30.4%

- have poor personal hygiene – 14.3%.

However, there were some positive views expressed with the following percentage of respondents agreeing that people with dementia:

- are able to participate in a wide variety of activities – 38.6%

- are a good source of wisdom – 37.7%

- can pass on valued traditions – 34.4%.

The results also indicate that there is an expectation by many in the community that if they receive a diagnosis of dementia they would feel a sense of shame or humiliation or experience depression or anxiety. Many were also afraid that a diagnosis would mean that they would be discriminated against both in the community and in the health sector. Alzheimer's Australia is committed to raising awareness about dementia and reducing the stigma and social isolation that often accompanies a diagnosis (Alzheimer's Australia 2012).

CHAPTER 19

The Language of Dementia

Sticks and stones will break my bones, but names will never hurt me.

(THE CHRISTIAN RECORDER, MARCH 1862)

Language and dementia

Changing the current disrespectful and disempowering language often used to refer to people with dementia will help remove discrimination, stigma and isolation. As far back as 2009, Alzheimer's Australia said in their *Dementia-friendly Language Position Paper 4*, which was updated in 2014:

> Language is a powerful tool. The words we use can strongly influence how others treat or view people with dementia. For example referring to people with dementia as 'sufferers' or as 'victims' implies that they are helpless. This not only strips people of their dignity and self-esteem, it reinforces inaccurate stereotypes and heightens the fear and stigma surrounding dementia.

Language is powerful and important in the discussions around providing person-centred care to people with dementia in a way that shows respect and dignity for the person. I still feel there is a very thin line between people with dementia being treated with dignity as opposed to being treated like morons, and I firmly believe nothing will change until we recognise it is imperative we all understand the human cost of dementia, and change the language we use about and referring to people with dementia.

Is language important?

- It defines the way others see us.
- It allows others to communicate with us.
- It defines the way we view ourselves.
- It allows us to communicate with others.
- It can impact stigma and discrimination.
- It can demean, devalue, disrespect and offend.

The time is now that people with dementia all over the world are standing up and speaking out about what is and isn't best for them, and this includes the language being used to refer to us. It is not a phenomenon, it is a basic human right, and as someone who is living with dementia, I have been advocating for a more respectful, empowering positive language for a long time. There is a long way still to go, and the language used about people with dementia, whilst it may not break my bones, can and does offend.

The language of dementia

The language of dementia is changing or evolving into one that is more acceptable to people with dementia. It may well be the key to a more person-centred approach to care and the key to reducing shame and stigma.

Until recently, the language of dementia has been decided by people without dementia. Not just family care partners, but care providers, nurses and doctors, people in the media, researchers and academics. Now people with dementia are speaking up and saying if it is acceptable. For the most part, it is not.

The current language being used by researchers, governments, the media, the acute hospital sector and in dementia and aged care is not aligned with language standards set by consumers as far back as 2008 (Alzheimer's Society of Ireland), DEEP and updated during Dementia Awareness Month by Alzheimer's Australia (2009, 2014) as part of its Dementia-friendly Communities resources.

Stigma towards people with dementia is a salient feature of their lived experience and language contributes significantly to this. The stigmatising, negative and disempowering language used in research about the very group researchers aim to improve outcomes for is not only disrespectful to people with dementia, but may prevent the timely translation of good research into better practice.

Reinforcing stereotypes

Our words do reflect our thoughts and feelings and can show respect or disrespect, and language is a powerful tool (Hughes, Louw and Sabat 2006). The words we use can strongly influence how others treat or view people with dementia. For example, referring to people with dementia as 'sufferers' or 'victims' implies that we are helpless, and this not only strips us of our dignity and self-esteem, it reinforces inaccurate stereotypes and heightens the fear and stigma surrounding dementia.

Society listened to other groups asking for the language used to refer to them to change to one they found more respectful. People with disAbilities quite reasonably expect not to be referred to as 'retards' or 'cripples', our gay community no longer accepts offensive, disrespectful or disempowering words about them and our Indigenous communities similarly have the same expectation and right to the use of empowering and respectful language, and one they have chosen, or at least been involved in advocating for.

The word dementia comes from the Latin meaning madness, so no wonder we struggle against the myths. Last year a State politician justified calling me 'demented', because, she said, technically I am! Although I told her I find that term very offensive, she stated she had a right to use it, and I was being overly pedantic, although I doubt if she would call an Indigenous Australian a 'black' or 'nigger', at least not to his or her face, or a person with a disAbility retarded, which was once the meaning of the word disabled.

The Google Online Dictionary defines dementia as 'a chronic or persistent disorder of the mental processes caused by brain disease or injury and marked by memory disorders, personality changes, and impaired reasoning'. The synonyms listed are: *mental illness, madness, insanity, derangement, lunacy, demented, dements, senile dementia, Alzheimer's, Alzheimer's disease.*

In contrast to dementia, disAbled is defined as '(persons) having a physical or mental condition that limits their movements, senses, or activities', and the synonyms listed are: *having a disAbility, wheelchair-using, paralysed.* Two years ago many of the following words were listed as synonyms for the word disAbility, but are now listed as words which are offensive and no longer appropriate to use: 'Offensive: retard, retarded, tard, handicapped, impaired, crip, cripple, lame.' I have this hope for the definition of dementia.

Communicating 'about' people with disAbilities

If you're communicating about disAbility issues or people with disAbilities here are a few golden rules to live by:

- Ask yourself if it's necessary to identify the person as having a disAbility. If you're preparing a document on community gardening in which a person with muscular dystrophy provided comment on the best type of trees to plant, their disAbility is irrelevant, as is dementia.

- Always put the person first. When describing someone with a disAbility they are not totally defined by their disAbility, such as in the phrase 'wheelchair bound'. Instead they are a 'person using a wheelchair, or wheelchair user'.

- Avoid using pitying or sensationalist terms. Most people with disAbilities don't see themselves as 'debilitated' or even 'inspiring' – they just see themselves as people like anyone else.

Will changing the model of care currently used in dementia change the narrative of dementia? I believe so, as the language of disAbility is already respectful, and has to some extent positively changed the way this group is seen in our community.

I think this speaks for itself. If we change the model of care to one that is supporting our disAbilities, we have a chance of empowering people to strive to live their pre-diagnosis lives, and to fight for their own wellbeing.

Language matters

We use the word 'disAbled' rather than retarded, because people with disAbilities started to speak up for themselves, and many found the word 'retarded' disrespectful…even though the dictionary definition once suggested it was appropriate.

No longer are 'sufferer', 'demented' or 'a vacant dement', as I sometimes still read, acceptable terms for people with dementia.

First and foremost, we are people, with names, living with dementia.

The term 'living with dementia' is also now only appropriate to use for the person diagnosed with dementia, the very people it affects more deeply, and the reality is that the person living with someone who is diagnosed with dementia is not living with dementia; they are living with someone diagnosed and living with dementia. But lately, I have changed my thinking on this a little…

There is often an almost angry refusal by many care partners to accept that they do not live with dementia, in the sense of being diagnosed with dementia and knowing what it is like to live with it.

> My mum, 88, is now in residential care. She has dementia; we have both lived with it for many years…

This daughter is not saying she is living with dementia; she is saying they have both lived with 'it' for many years. There is a subtle difference; if you think of dementia as we do in my house, and that 'it' is the third person in the threesome, it could be seen as us both living with 'it'. And we call this troublesome threesome the Three Stooges, and have even named 'it', Larry!

It sounds more acceptable than the family care partners who insist they are living with dementia themselves, even though they are care partners, and not the person diagnosed. Stated this way, they cannot be living with dementia as they are not diagnosed with it. But they are living with 'it', this third 'person' in the relationship, albeit as care partners and not diagnosed with 'it'.

So, on the topic of language, I am, as I imagine everyone is, learning more and seeing things differently almost every day. Although I still believe that unless you have dementia you do not know what it is like to live with it, in the same way as unless you have been through childbirth you do not know what that is like to give birth to a baby.

Language in the workforce

The most fundamental skills required in any organisation are language, literacy and numeracy, and these enable us to:

- process information
- communicate effectively
- contribute to productivity and performance
- enjoy socialisation and team building and our general ability to enjoy our job and work environment
- build confidence
- build the ability to adapt to our changing environments.

Language, literacy and numeracy (LLN) enable us to process information, communicate effectively and contribute to productivity and performance, as well as socialisation, team building and our general ability to enjoy our job and work environment. These skills also arm us with confidence and the ability to adapt to our changing environments.

Therefore, in the workforce, it is critical that workers have the knowledge to recognise when a person with dementia needs assistance with language, literary or numeracy and adjust their care and education accordingly.

This surely applies to how health care staff deliver care to people with dementia, as our impairments should require that staff have knowledge in how to assist with our impairments. Unfortunately, I have more often seen impairments being viewed as 'difficult behaviours', which are then treated with restraint of some kind, rather than seen as impairments to the person's ability to communicate.

I find it curious that speech pathologists are rarely included in the care plans of people with dementia, at least in Australia, especially considering our language and speech impairments, and their expertise in this area. It is definitely food for thought.

Let's hope also that those people caring for people with dementia will consider the impairments we have in language, literacy and numeracy, and assist us with better strategies to manage them, rather than 'treat' us with drugs or other forms of restraint or insults. It might appear funny not knowing how to use a biro, but the frustration of not being able to do a simple task like that would be very annoying! I know, and although most times I still know how to use a biro, I cannot always remember how to sign my name, and many other simple tasks have become difficult, or impossible.

In the milieu of people with dementia, this is important. If we cannot enjoy nor have the ability to continue with good language, literacy and numeracy, then our experience of happiness and wellbeing is impaired. Of course we will display 'challenging behaviours' if no-one bothers to understand us, or our needs.

When people with dementia have reduced or impaired language abilities, then it is up to others to learn how to communicate with them, not the other way around. If challenging behaviours become part of the experience, then it is more likely due to not being able to express things like pain, poor-tasting food, being bored, than it is the fault of the dementia.

If we continue to behave in challenging ways, then others need to change something, not us, and using physical or chemical restraint is not the answer, but rather a blatant abuse of our human right to be understood and cared for the best way possible.

Language and the media

- The media continues to stigmatise and labels us with devaluing and negative language.

- Journalists mostly refuse to engage in debate with people with dementia regarding respectful language.

- Many in the media still refuse to view the word suffering in the same way they view the word retarded.

- Most ignore the latest language guidelines.

As the editor of an international advocacy and support group of, by and for people with dementia, I read or am referred to many articles in the media about dementia. Most of them require a comment from people living with dementia, in order to either reclaim our human rights, to request the same respect offered to everyone else in the community, or to complain about either the misconceptions and myths the articles portray, due to the ignorance of those without dementia, or the biases and prejudices of a few.

After over four years of being told by people in the media that I had no right to be offended by terms such as 'sufferer', since September 2014 I have had five journalists (yes, so far *only* five) agree I (we) do have a right to be offended, that they have a responsibility to be respectful on our terms, not theirs, and then who have actually bothered to change their words as a result of my communication with them. I send up to five emails or messages most weeks to journalists and others in the media, asking them to refer to the latest language guidelines. Most don't even bother to respond, but of those that do, they always agree using the words retard or retarded are disrespectful… Never any arguments there!

Most people believe that if a word or term is in the public domain, and a group of people find it offensive, then we do have the right to ask others to stop using it, in the same way we – and they – would *never* refer to a person with an intellectual or physical disAbility as a retard or retarded any more. Not because they are not retarded, as technically they are, but because this group of people find it offensive. I often call myself retarded to make a point, and people are horrified I would refer to myself that way, and often, these same people are then aggressive in their right to offend me and other people living with dementia by calling us victims, sufferers or demented or, worse, demented sufferers.

Suffering from vs diagnosed with?

I have written extensively a number of times about language and dementia, including this:

> Does 'I am suffering from…dementia, arthritis, cancer or Multiple Sclerosis' sound more negative and less empowering than 'I am diagnosed with…'? Whilst the term suffering may technically be 'correct', I fail to see how anyone could not see it is not negative and disempowering.[1]

1 http://kateswaffer.com/2014/05/26/diagnosed-with-vs-suffering-from-dementia

We [people with dementia] are also not 'not all there' or 'fading away'; we are still here, and we still have feelings and opinions and rights. Some of us may 'suffer' from dementia or other diseases some or all of the time, but that does not necessarily make us all *sufferers*.

The media spoon-feeds the public, and has a responsibility to feed it the truth, with respect for all of those it portrays. This includes people with dementia.

Language in research

The language in research continues to label us negatively, further exacerbating the stigma, isolation, shame and discrimination. This may well be part of what is effecting knowledge translation into better practice.

I have explored stigma in the literature, looking at it in a new way by questioning whether the researchers exacerbate stigma, even though their intent is to promote positive change. Considering the lack of inclusion of people with dementia in the cohorts being studied, it is still very much 'about them, without them', which cannot give a true picture of the issues at hand for this particular group, and simply serves to reinforce the stigma. Caregiver stigma has been explored often (Dean 2011a; Mackenzie 2006; Phillipson *et al.* 2012; Werner *et al.* 2012) but very little on the stigma as experienced directly by people with dementia.

No longer can this expertise be ignored as people with dementia are the experts through the lived experience, and not including them in research not only stigmatises them, but it hinders the validity of the research. This is important as much of the published research is biased through the use of family care partners as the main cohort group, or having them in attendance when people with dementia are interviewed, and so the care partner voice remains the main voice in the stigma research.

There is a significant body of evidence to draw upon, and the literature appears to show more positive attitudes. However, this may be a socially acceptable veneer covering up the embedded and unconscious negative attitudes that drive human behaviour, expressed as stigma and discrimination.

Language in health care

- Medical benefits require the use of certain labels to provide certain payments.

- Health care workers continue to use negative labels that dehumanise people with dementia.

- This continues to stigmatise people with dementia.

The language being used to refer to people with dementia in the health sector needs to change. Providing person-centred care simply will not happen until the language about us is respectful, and stops labelling us as 'challenging behaviours', or worse. We are people, not behaviours, and, more often than not, a behaviour is a form of communicating a need or want, no more no less, and the person who is not disAbled needs to learn how to communicate with us, not restrain us to 'manage' us.

Learning a new language

South Australian MP Kelly Vincent says when communicating with people with disAbilities, they are the experts; so too are those people diagnosed with dementia.

We would not hesitate to consider the communication needs of a child or a person with a speech disAbility and yet this is frequently not the case for people with dementia. Karen Fossum (2003) wrote: 'When your child is no longer a child, you will have to find a new language.'

That is not to say people with dementia wish to be spoken to like we are children, but rather that the same amount of effort and respect is placed on learning to communicate with us as our needs change.

This surely applies to how health care staff deliver care to people with dementia, as our impairments should require that staff know how to assist with our impairments. Unfortunately, I have more often seen impairments regarded as 'difficult behaviours', which are then treated with restraint of some kind, rather than seen as impairments to the person's ability to communicate.

Of course we will display 'challenging behaviours' if no-one bothers to understand our frustrations, or our needs.

When people with dementia have reduced or impaired language abilities, then it is up to others to learn how to communicate with them, not the other way around. If challenging behaviours become part of the experience, it is more likely due to the person not being able to express things like pain, dissatisfaction with poor-tasting food or being bored, than it is the fault of the person's dementia.

If we continue to behave in challenging ways, then others need to change something, not us. Using physical or chemical restraint is not the answer, but rather a blatant abuse of our human right to be understood and cared for in the best way possible.

It is also a human right for people with dementia, many of whom have speech impairments and language difficulties, to expect the provision of speech pathologists to provide care and assistance to maintain language for as long as possible. So far, this allied health specialist is missing in action in the dementia sector, and I have never seen or heard of one being employed to assist people with dementia, other than the one I use, engaged privately.

Language and stigma

Language is important. It not only defines how people see us but ultimately how we view ourselves. It allows us to communicate with others, and can impact stigma and discrimination. It has the potential to promote and empower, enable and increase self-esteem, and encourage one's ability to self-help and self-advocate. Or it can demean, devalue, disrespect and offend those we refer to.

Language affects the experience of stigma. The phrase 'sticks and stones may break my bones but words will never hurt me', in my experience of living with dementia and listening to the way we are referred to and spoken about, is wrong. They do hurt me and the use of offensive and demeaning labels and language simply intensifies the shame and stigma we already feel.

Family care partners continue to write and speak about us as sufferers; I claim it is they who are suffering, far more than us, and my husband agrees with me.

Considering the lack of inclusion of people with dementia in the cohorts being studied, it is still very much 'about them, without them', which cannot give a true picture of the issues at hand for this particular group, and simply serves to reinforce the stigma.

Language, inclusion and providing dementia-friendly communities are important in the reduction of stigma, and without positive change, stigma will continue to be a significant burden on people with dementia.

Does language matter?

Yes, language does matter; at least to the person or group of people it might offend.

As in the section above, consider the phrase '*suffering from*' dementia vs '*diagnosed with*' dementia. The first one is negative and disempowering. 'Demented' is also no longer an acceptable term for people with dementia. And I repeat, first and foremost we are people, with feelings and names and identities, living with dementia.

When talking about language and difference – language and how it makes us think about people and act towards them has a practical impact on the way members of our community treat those of us we see as being different. In the past, and now, much of the language used to refer to people with disAbility or impairment and life-limiting disease has been developed by others such as researchers or clinicians.

It can be argued that this medicalised approach has led to most of us thinking about the impairment or disease – the condition – before the person and this may well be one of the barriers to the provision of person-centred care. It's my belief that this sort of approach leads to a sense of treating people as 'other', or 'us and them'.

You can argue that this is at the heart of discrimination and helps create a sense, or reality, of fractured community. A more recent move has been to try to see the person first and then the condition, but negative disrespectful language can hold this back.

Speaking up

We are all part of a contiguous community, we all live here, we are all people and we all need to consider each other as people – not cases, subjects or conditions. In today's thinking, those of us who belong to an identifiable group have advocated for the right, capacity, ability, 'permission' to identify themselves, speak for themselves and promote the language that is used about us.

While no individual in any identifiable group can be said to be the single voice of that group, it remains the right of that group as a community to have a voice to speak about how it is that the 'rest of us' speak about them – therein lies empowerment.

Changing the current disrespectful and disempowering language will help to remove the discrimination, stigma and isolation, and will help others see that many people with dementia are still very capable of contributing positively. As we have not been active in our own advocacy until recently, it is not yet the norm, and this affects how people view and treat us.

It is a very recent phenomenon that people with dementia are included in the conversations that are about them. Sadly, staying engaged means many people with dementia are accused of lying about their diagnosis. Personally I prefer to ignore these doubters and continue to strive to live beyond dementia; it comes from the stigma still very present, and from the myths and ignorance still in the community and health and dementia care sectors.

It is clear from the numbers of people with dementia who are standing up and speaking out as advocates that there is still a good life to live even after a diagnosis of dementia. We do not have to accept the Prescribed Disengagement®

and give up our pre-diagnosis lives. As I have written previously (Swaffer 2014a, 2014b, 2015), I recommend to everyone who has been diagnosed with dementia and who has accepted the prescription of disengagement, to ignore this well-meaning but negative advice, and re-invest in life.

People can live beyond dementia but the language used about them needs to be normal, inclusive, jargon-free, non-elitist, clear, straightforward, non-judgemental and centre on the person, not the disease or social care system, or language trends that come and go. It is absolutely the time for governments, the media, the health care sector, researchers and the community at large to reconsider the way they refer to us and speak about us, and to listen to our request for something as simple as language that people with dementia agree is respectful.

Finally, I developed this slide in 2014, which began with 17 things, and then after much 'consultation' via my blog, I adjusted it and added three more points. My next book is to be based on this list, with a chapter for each point, first of why not to do or say these things, and then what the more respectful alternatives are.

20 ways to more positively support a person with dementia

1 Don't say, 'But you don't look or sound like you have dementia'.

2 Don't tell us we are wrong.

3 Don't argue with us over trivial things.

4 Don't say 'remember when…'

5   Don't call us 'sufferers' or 'victims'.

6   Don't say we are 'demented', 'demented sufferers', 'fading away', 'disappearing', have a 'dementing illness', an 'empty shell', or 'not all there'.

7   Don't say you are 'living with dementia' unless you are diagnosed with dementia.

8   Don't remind us of the death of a loved one or pet.

9   Don't blame the person for the changes in behaviour or personality.

10 Don't assume we do not understand you.

11 We have a form of dementia, not an 'affliction'.

12 Don't call me 'honey', 'love' or anything other than my preferred name.

13 Don't refer to us as 'aggressives', 'wanderers', 'poor feeders', 'wetters', 'non-communicators' or as 'obstructive' – we are still human beings. Don't assume we can't feel pain just because we may not be able to tell you about it.

14 Don't assume because we can't tell you, your words or actions don't hurt our feelings.

15 Don't assume I can't answer for myself.

16 Don't talk about me to someone else, in front of me.

17 Don't assume we can't communicate even if we can't speak.

18 Don't say, 'but I've just told you that' or 'you've asked me that already'.

19 Don't think we can't feel pain, or emotions.

20 Don't assume anything, or that I don't understand just because I am silent.

Please also consider downloading, and embracing in your home or workplace, the latest Alzheimer's Australia *Dementia Language Guidelines*, updated in 2014.[2]

I wrote the list of 20 things not to do or say to a person with dementia in the hope that it might positively impact the life of even one more person living with dementia. If this happens, it does not matter how many people with dementia disagreed with me.

The list was not written to upset or criticise care partners, but to help them understand that making a few changes to the way they are when they are around people with dementia might improve our experience of dementia and therefore make their job easier.

It was only ever written up to try to reduce the 'burden' so many tell us we are to them. But perhaps my directness is too blunt, and needs more discussion, and a second book on why not to do or say these things, and what the alternative is, is in progress. Dementia has encouraged me to be more direct than I was before, it has reduced my shyness and increased my willingness to discuss the difficult topics. Unfortunately, that may come across as unkind or critical, when it is not meant to be. It may also be that I am more direct than I mean to be, because if the inner frustration I

---

2   https://fightdementia.org.au/sites/default/files/NATIONAL/documents/ language-guidelines-full.pdf

continue to feel that the voices of people with dementia are mostly still being ignored, and there is, after so many years of 'about us, without us', still such a long way to go.

CHAPTER 20

Dementia and Word Finding

The creator of *Moving Your Soul*,[1] one of the few blogs by and for care partners of people with dementia I really respect and follow, asked me to reply to a question from one of their blog followers: 'I would like to know about your symptoms at the beginning of your process before the diagnosis of dementia'. It started me thinking…and revisiting this time in my life, and the impact of not being able to find the right word or words.

Part of my response to Susana was to add a quote I had written soon after diagnosis:

> My high functioning mind has slipped away, sometimes showing itself like a ghost, trying to tease me into believing it will be okay, but now outside of my reach. My thoughts fly around inside my head like helium balloons high inside an auditorium, also out of my reach.

What happens when people with dementia can't find the right words or when our thought processes become confused and muddled? To begin with we worry, and struggle with feelings of humiliation and a loss of dignity. We feel embarrassed and ashamed. We feel frustrated and

---

1   www.movingyoursoul.com/es/author/movingyoursoul

annoyed. And I still regularly wonder, 'What the hell happened to my brain?'

Memory is like a stack of china. If you pull a plate from the middle of the stack, it comes crashing down. If others constantly try to hurry us or speak for us or help to remind us what they think we are trying to remember and say, that is when our words come tumbling down. Memories are also a bit like a stack of books. The books are there; sometimes we can't locate them, nor remember what we have read. Words are quite often somewhere inside our head but often we can't find them, but much more than the occasional walking into the next room and forgetting what we went for.

The challenge for us, whilst we still have insight, is the time it takes, or the growing frustration of not being able to find the right word. For me, I am also speaking 'back to front' if I don't take time, e.g. I will say 'go left', when I mean 'go right'. It is also the speed of which a thought disappears, before you have grasped it which makes it difficult to communicate, and challenging to live with.

My language is also becoming more generic, as everything is often being called 'this' or 'that' and the struggle we have in my home to work out what the hell this or that actually means is not always fun. Mostly, though, we do try to laugh about it.

Playing charades might help, but only if your family and friends know you really well!

CHAPTER 21 ———————————————————

Employment and Dementia

Employers are not in most cases, and definitely were not in my personal experience, what kept me from remaining in paid work after my diagnosis. Prescribed Disengagement® was the main culprit. Being told to give up life as I knew it, and get acquainted with aged care and to prepare for death, was the problem. It removed my sense of hope for a future, and even the idea that with reasonable adjustments, I may be able to stay at work after my driving licence was revoked. Sure, my employer at the time did not encourage, or even suggest I might be able to remain employed, but if I had thought I might be able to live beyond dementia with supports for the disAbilities, at least for a while, then I would not have given up work so easily.

The issue of employment currently is more likely to affect people with younger onset dementia, but as many older people are choosing to work beyond the current retirement age, this may change.

Most people with dementia live in the community, and with support, many people with dementia are able to remain active and participate in many of the same activities they did before they received a diagnosis, including paid work. There are some people diagnosed with dementia that may appear to have no external symptoms at all, but who still may require assistance.

If a worker experiences a stroke or head injury employers have a legal obligation to provide them with reasonable support to return to work, and currently, there is usually high intent to do so. This is not yet the case for people with dementia, as we are still struggling with the myth that you can only die from dementia, not live with it positively.

Whilst people with dementia still have capacity and abilities, and also wish to remain employed, every effort must be made to support them with reasonable adjustments to allow them to continue working for as long as they may wish to remain employed.

On the other hand, even if they are still capable, not everyone wants to keep working after the diagnosis of dementia or any other terminal illness.

Some people just want to get their affairs in order, and then start to tick things off of their bucket lists. That's okay too, and totally optional, depending on the individual, and also the type of dementia. There are a few where prognosis is grim, and progression, even with non-pharmacological interventions, will happen quickly. Some employees may prefer not to remain employed; this is a very individual choice, and furthermore in some cases even where an employer provides a 'reasonable adjustment' the person with dementia may not be able to remain employed.

I am not a lawyer, or consultant on this area, and therefore this is not legal advice for either the employer or an employee with dementia. However well-informed, this is about my experiences, and my thoughts and opinions on the topic. For anyone who wants to remain at their place of employment, I would suggest you seek advice, and for all workplace relations and legal advice you should always seek professional legal consultation.

People with dementia have rights in relation to employment

I write this next section from the Australian perspective, but always suggest you seek legal consultation for your own situation. Some of the research I have done on the topic may either be wrong through misinterpretation, or legislation may have changed.

However, any person who has a disAbility, mental health or medical condition (including dementia) which impacts on their work is eligible for disability services such as *auxiliary aids*, meaning equipment (other than a palliative or therapeutic device) that provides assistance to a person with a disAbility to alleviate the effect of the disAbility (Disability Discrimination Act 1992).

A person's disAbility may require supporting documentation from the employee's treating practitioner (e.g. doctor, neurologist, psychologist, psychiatrist) to determine eligibility, but support for disabilities cannot legally be denied. In Part 2 – Prohibition of disability discrimination, Division 1 – Discrimination in work, 15. Discrimination in employment (1) 'It is unlawful for an employer or a person acting or purporting to act on behalf of an employer to discriminate against a person on the ground of the other person's disAbility or a disAbility of any of that other person's associate…'

People with dementia may wish to remain employed

As an employee with dementia, if you have capacity, and are capable of fulfilling your current role, or can do so with reasonable adjustments, you have a right to remain employed, if you so wish.

As an employer, the important point to remember is it is a person's legal right to remain employed, and to expect support to 'reasonable adjustments' providing this does not include adjustments which would impose an unjustifiable hardship on the employer (in the case of adjustments to enable a person to perform the inherent requirements of a job) or which would be unreasonable.

There will be circumstances where the employer might say that the person with dementia is unable to meet the requirements of the job even with reasonable adjustments; it is important to acknowledge that in some cases even with 'reasonable adjustment' a person with dementia may not be able to remain employed.

It is not discrimination under the Disability Discrimination Act to:

- fail or refuse to employ a person for a job, or fail or refuse to transfer or promote the person to a job

- terminate a person's employment in a job.

But, this is only if:

- the person is unable, or would be unable, to perform the inherent requirements of that job, and

- this inability cannot be remedied by making a reasonable adjustment.

The increasing number of people with dementia will mean this will only become more of an issue. The rights of people with disAbilities, including people with dementia, mean that employers have a duty to assist and ensure this can happen for those people who might wish to remain employed, and where reasonable adjustments can be made.

Currently, the economic cost of dementia to younger people diagnosed with it is significant, as they are usually people with children to support, and households to maintain, often including rent or a mortgage. If it is possible, with the appropriate support for disAbilities, to remain employed, there are benefits not only to the individuals, but their families, the health care sector and society as a whole. It also supports the reduction of stigma, discrimination, isolation and reduces the misperceptions others have about dementia.

It was very encouraging that the World Alzheimer's Report 2015 discussed our right to remain employed, and also our rights to be employed. I was delighted to see two vacancies at a UK organisation advertised on Twitter, where one of the criteria was to have a diagnosis of dementia. In the dementia-friendly communities initiatives and campaigns, people with dementia are the perfect people to employ, in the same way we would employ an IT expert for our companies' IT, and Indigenous or gay people if we were working towards Indigenous- or gay-friendly communities. It would definitely not be about them, without them, as it currently is with us.

Supporting disAbilities

It is important to remember that the disAbilities of a person with dementia may be supported in the same way as any other disAbled person. These may include support for learning or other cognitive disAbilities, as well as visual, hearing, mobility or other physical disAbilities. The following is a list of disAbilities, followed by a list of strategies and resources. Both lists may not cover every disAbility or possible support. Research shows there is a much higher chance of successfully supporting a person with dementia to remain employed and to successfully use

Assisted Technology or other supports if introduced to them at an earlier stage of dementia.

The following is a list of some disAbilities caused by the symptoms of cognitive impairment or dementia, which can be well supported to maintain some level of functioning. I proved this at the University of South Australia, and then again in 2014 receiving disability support from the University of Wollongong.

- Dyslexia.

- Word finding or understanding, or changes in comprehension abilities.

- Vision impairment.

- Spatial or other sight impairment affecting mobility.

- Hearing impairment.

- Learning difficulties that require support.

- Memory impairment, e.g. retention of new information.

- Motivation may be lower at times.

- Organisation and planning abilities may be impaired.

- Reduced attention span, difficulty starting or maintaining activities; don't assume the worker is tired, lazy or disinterested but rather encourage and support.

- Judgement and reasoning changes.

- Loss of insight and some social skills.

Strategies to support the disAbilities of cognitive impairment/dementia

Strategies to support the disAbilities of cognitive impairment or dementia can include Assisted Technology (AT). AT is any product or piece of equipment used to maintain or improve the functional capabilities of people with disAbilities. Incorporating AT for employees with dementia into the workplace can be useful for employees who are experiencing disAbilities of dementia. There are other more simple strategies, as well as dementia enabling office and building design, including clear signage.

The following is a list of AT, support software and other strategies, although not exhaustive as new AT is being developed all the time:

- Support for acquired dyslexia. This may include simple things like additional software for spelling, or providing the minutes of meetings as a Word document as well as having them recorded.

- Time management support.

- Using email or notes to record meetings, i.e. if you have a conversation, it might assist the person with dementia if to follow it up with a précis of what has been discussed or requested; if it is via email, then the person (and you) automatically has a record of the conversation.

- Adaptive technology, software and equipment, for example:

  » Up-to-date computer with USB ports on the front to allow easy plug-in of headphones and other equipment.

» 20" large-screen LCD monitor that is easily adjustable on a swing arm so that it can be positioned to suit a range of users.

» A4 scanner allowing hard copy material to be converted into electronic text, so that it can be used with the specialised software and enlarged or read from the screen.

» A3/A4 printer allowing material to be easily printed in enlarged text.

» Dragon Naturally Speaking speech recognition software. This software provides users with the ability to write essays and emails and even explore the web by voice command. It can be very useful for students who have difficulty working at a keyboard or using text. Students with a range of disAbilities such as arthritis, RSI or learning disAbilities may find this a valuable resource.

» Zoomtext software provides text magnification along with screen reading so that users can listen to the material which appears on the screen. This product is designed especially for people with vision impairment.

» Read & Write software is designed for use by people who have a learning disAbility. It provides features such as enhanced spelling and grammar checking, word prediction and screen reading in an easy to use package.

» Spectronics.

- Word finding or understanding, or changes in comprehension abilities can be supported with the use of visual aids, and alternatives such as audio or video files.

- Vision impairment can be supported with computer software for screen enlargement; audio aids may also assist.

- Spatial or other sight impairment affecting mobility can be supported with things such as hand rails and following enabling environment design principles.

- Hearing impairments can be supported with visual aids.

- Learning and/or memory impairment can be supported with electronic reminders, as well as having a support person at work to mentor and buddy.

- Additional time may be required to complete tasks.

- Mobility support and aids, e.g. walking sticks, offer a person support with spatial and visual depth perceptions problems.

- Hearing aids, e.g. using microphones for speakers during meetings.

- Prior to and during meetings:

  » Staff with dementia may need to be able to ask questions or comment as they think of them, rather than be asked to wait as they may not always be able to 'hold that thought'.

  » Provide meeting minutes in a verbal format, e.g. podcast or a simple set of spoken minutes.

» Provide reading material in advance of meetings.

» All meeting papers should be sent as early as possible.

» Papers should be presented in a clear, organised and numbered manner in the folder.

» Feedback can be provided from members in writing prior to the meeting if they wish to do so. This feedback can then either be distributed to other members for consideration prior to the meeting or presented at the meeting by the member, another member or chair.

• Natural supports can easily be provided; this simply means support in a workplace can be assistance through relationships, buddies or mentors, as well as interactions that allow the person with dementia to work in a job of their choice in ways similar to other employees.

Language and education about dementia

These are two very important steps in supporting a person with dementia in their workplace. It is important to remember the language you use can be inclusive and respectful, or it can be exclusive, demeaning and disrespectful. This is part of being dementia-friendly, and includes ensuring your staff all refer to the recently updated Alzheimer's Australia Dementia Language Guidelines 2014.[1]

---

1   https://fightdementia.org.au/sites/default/files/full%20language%20 guidelines%20final.pdf

Improve the work environment for people with dementia

There are some simple steps that can be taken to create a more dementia-friendly work environment. The design principles of dementia-enabling environments are an important tool, and although a building may not be able to be renovated to meet their guidelines, many simple steps can be taken within the work space to improve it. This includes things like improving the lighting in all areas, adding hand rails, ensuring all signs are large, and clear, with black text on white background. Professor Richard Fleming from the University of Wollongong is one of the world leaders in this area, and I recommend you go to the Dementia Enabling Environments Project for further information.[2]

Respect and communication

Respect, kindness, patience, common sense, and using good communication skills are simple steps to support a person living with the disAbilties of dementia. Learning to communicate with a person with language or cognitive impairment is as important as learning to communicate with someone who has lost their speech after a stroke or some other disAbling condition. It is not the person's fault, and it is up to others without disAbilities to make the time, and effort to learn about the disease, and how to best communicate.

Finally, I believe any time off during the diagnostic process should be supported with sick leave in the same way you would if the person had been diagnosed with another terminal illness such as cancer. It is no reason to have to resign.

2   www.enablingenvironments.com.au

External organisations and services supporting disAbilities in Australia

(Please search for similar organisations in your own country.)

- Employee Assistance Program
- Australian Human Rights Commission
- Australian Human Rights Commission – Mental Health in the Workplace

External disAbility services

- Blind Welfare Association
- Guide Dogs Australia
- Royal Society for the Blind
- Health Insite
- Disability Information and Resource Centre Inc (DIRC)
- Deaf CanDo

Federal and state legislation

- Australian Human Rights Commission Act 1986
- Disability Discrimination Act 1992
- Age Discrimination Act 2004
- Racial Discrimination Act 1975
- Sex Discrimination Act 1984

Driving and Dementia

HER SYMBOL OF INDEPENDENCE

She sat in the Ute aged seven
Atop three pillows
Just so she could see to drive
The joy of this freedom
Like wind in her nostrils
Or the salty fresh sea breeze
This symbol of independence
She felt would never end...

(KATE SWAFFER 2015)

Driving is a powerful symbol of competence and independence, and is a routine part of one's adult life. It is not a human right.

As a person living with a diagnosis of dementia, I have a very contentious view about driving and dementia. Let me start by redefining dementia, simply because the definition is significant when thinking about my rationale regarding driving and dementia.

'Dementia affects thinking, behaviour and the ability to perform everyday tasks. Brain function is affected enough to interfere with the person's normal social or working life' (Alzheimer's Australia 2013). It can be seen as the gradual deterioration of functioning, such as thinking, concentration, memory, and judgement, which affects a person's ability to perform normal daily activities. The Mayo Clinic says: 'Memory loss generally occurs in dementia, but memory loss alone doesn't mean you have dementia. Dementia indicates problems with at least two brain functions, such as memory loss and impaired judgment or language' (2013).

Driving is a risky business. It demands focused concentration, quick reaction times, good judgement, and efficient problem-solving skills, as well as alertness and perception. At the core of this discussion are the safety of the driver, and the safety of others. The majority of us commenced driving aged 16 and not until we achieve older age are we ever re-assessed for safety or fitness to drive, without a known health issue. We do not have to undertake a single written test, or practical skills test, or a defensive driving course at any time after our licence is granted.

People with dementia eventually lose these abilities and skills, but unfortunately many people with dementia do not recognise these losses when they happen, or if they do, the stress of losing their independence is so high, they lie about their driving ability. Many family care partners also lie about their partner's driving abilities, and on top of that doctors are also loath to confront the issue, for a number of reasons, not least because it may prevent the person from attending to other health needs.

Signs that dementia may be affecting driving abilities

- Returning from a habitual drive later than usual.
- An increased number of dents and scratches on the car.
- Forgetting how to get to and from familiar places.

- Going out in the car, then getting a taxi home, forgetting you had gone out in the car.

- Losing the car in a places like a car park.

- Getting lost.

- Failing to observe traffic signs.

- Going down one-way streets the wrong direction.

- Making slow or poor decisions in traffic.

- Slow reaction times.

- Driving at inappropriate speeds, too slow or too fast.

- Misjudging speed, distance or turns.

- Becoming angry, stressed, agitated or confused while driving.

- Hitting kerbs.

- Misjudging car parking.

- Poor lane control.

- Making errors at intersections.

- Confusing the brake and accelerator pedals.

Whilst driving a motor vehicle is not as complex as flying a plane, this does seem unsafe. With a pilot's licence, the pilot has to have a bi-annual flight review/test, and full medical examinations, which escalate after the age of 40 (Civil Aviation Safety Authority 2013). It includes eyesight, hearing, urine checks for diabetes, and ECG; they must also be done if they have not flown in the previous three months, done at least three take-offs circuits and landings, before taking any passengers up. On the other hand, in Australia we are legally able to get a driver's licence at age 16, which we renew by paying money and a new photo. We are then considered safe to drive until our health assessments start at age 70, although this is different depending on what state in Australia you live in, and in which country you live.

Aged 50 and with a diagnosis of younger onset dementia, I had my driver's licence revoked after failing a practical assessment. My neurologist and neuropsychologist thought I would pass. I thought I would probably pass. I failed, with a very low score of 35 per cent, a shock to them, and an even greater shock to me. It has impacted my independence and self-esteem, and, of course, my ability to get around.

It is one of the most emotionally debilitating aspects of dementia. The emotional and financial impact of surrendering or having your driver's licence revoked is significant, and many of the issues are not obvious, especially to others.

The toll of having my driver's licence revoked includes the following:

- significant loss and grief – it feels like a death; in fact, for me, it was perhaps worse than the diagnosis of dementia

- loss of independence

- loss of control

- loss of independent 'mobility'

- loss of privacy

- lowers self-esteem and self-worth

- feelings of incompetence

- loss of social equality

- increased stigma

- increased discrimination

- increased isolation

- increased loneliness

- increased guilt

- the guilt then increases the sadness

- inability to be independent and self-sufficient

- tension and anxiety relying on others

- reduced family income; loss of work hours for partner to provide transport

- buses and taxis can be too difficult for people with dementia to negotiate

- sense of wellbeing significantly impaired

- increased sense of being a burden.

Since relying on others for transport, I have come to realise many people still licensed to drive are less able to drive than I was! When my father-in-law who had Lewy body dementia was unsafe driving, it took us 18 months to get his doctor to take it seriously, and a threat of advising the insurance company if he had an accident that the doctor should be held accountable, for him to take any notice. Dad was driving around roundabouts the wrong way, stopping suddenly on a highway, in very unsafe places, driving on the wrong wide of the road (yes, sometimes with grandchildren in the car), and having numerous small accidents, but no amount of suggesting his licence be taken away, or he be re-assessed as fit to drive made any difference. The doctor was protective of him, and said many times he did not want to take away his independence. Dad always told the doctor he felt safe driving! Odenheimer (2006) reports, 'because of the emotional nature of the topic of driving, many physicians are reluctant to broach the participant with their patients'.

Currently in Australia, a diagnosis of dementia is not sufficient reason for the revoking of a person's driver's licence, and cognitive and physical abilities are not the only markers of safe driving. Professor Kaarin Anstey, in her model of factors enabling safe driving behaviour, says the following features are required for safe driving, including for people with a diagnosis of dementia: driving behaviour, capacity to drive safely, self-monitoring and beliefs about driving capacity, cognition, vision and physical functioning (Anstey *et al.* 2005). I would argue against this, and suggest a diagnosis of dementia impacts safe driving, because our ability to accurately (and honestly) self-monitor, our beliefs about our driving capacity and at least two markers, for example cognition, concentration or judgement, have been clinically identified. They have to be, for us to have a confirmed diagnosis of dementia!

The Austroads and the National Transport Commission revised the *Assessing Fitness to Drive Guidelines* in 2012, and they contain nationally agreed medical standards for the purposes of driver licensing, but is this enough? There are limited resources for testing drivers for safety, and the variance in laws and the ways in which people with dementia are tested for safety between states and territories is high. The cost of assessing fitness to drive is high, and borne entirely by the person with dementia; the required numbers of appropriately trained assessors are not yet available. The variations in states make it unsafe, as drivers are not limited by borders.

The Survey of Disability, Ageing and Care partners (SDAC) reported that 84 per cent of people with dementia had a profound level of limitation in core activities, while an additional 9 per cent had a severe level of limitation (ABS 2010). As a person with a diagnosis of dementia, this seems at odds with the advocacy of our rights to continue to drive, even with a conditional licence. In an investigation into 'The effects of Alzheimer's disease and mild cognitive impairment on driving ability', Fritelli *et al.* (2009) found results adding to the growing body of evidence that driving performance decreases even with mild cognitive impairment in AD.

I have anecdotal evidence of the test given to many people with younger onset dementia being a simple drive around the block, because they look young, fit and healthy. I also have a significant amount of anecdotal evidence of drivers who are creative with the law, and their self-assessment, who say to me they know they are unsafe, but rely on looking fit and healthy, and saying the right thing to their doctor. I know of older couples who support each other through unsafe driving, for example, one manages the gearstick because the driver cannot remember how to. They both report to their doctor the driver is safe.

We all know to drive under the influence of alcohol of drugs is illegal. During my 'good' moments, I am probably safe to drive, but the issue is, I cannot predict when this will change, and when the symptoms of dementia are in fuller flight; in this way it is similar to being under the influence of alcohol, but with no warning. One blog follower with dementia said this:

> Due to our brains ceasing to function as they did, I gave up my license immediately after my diagnosis. I knew I was a risk and could cause harm to others. With my losing focus and having mental lapses…that's a sure sign that the brain isn't doing its job? … I strongly speak out to others with dementia about what they are doing and they may cause

serious injury to others, apart from the possibility of invalid insurance.

The greatest issues for me personally are the burden I feel to others and the initial guilt which has turned into sadness for not being able to transport children, elderly parents, or meeting up with friends. And I do very much miss the spontaneity of being in control of my own transport. I would still argue, based on the definition of dementia, people with dementia are simply not safe to drive a vehicle averaging a weight of 1.5 tonnes, with a speed capability of 100+ km per hour, under any circumstance.

People with dementia do still have a responsibility to regard the safety of others, and if we lose the insight for this, then others should and must step in. I also know my opinion on driving and dementia is out of step with what some research, most professionals and people with dementia believe about driving, but I remain firm in my belief.

The notion that it is still safe to drive, when one's cognitive abilities are impaired to the point of a diagnosis of dementia, to me, flies in the face of simple common sense, but I realise governments are not ready or willing to afford the alternatives.

CHAPTER 23

Family Care Partners or BUBs (Back-Up Brains)

Dementia care is caring for people
Who often do not know they need care,
And don't want to be in care;
No wonder they may become angry and upset!

(KATE SWAFFER 2008)

Back-Up Brain (BUB)

The topic of what to call the family member, partner or friend who is supporting the person with dementia is fraught with danger, but to refer to them as a care partner not only strips them of their identity and from other important roles, it places a 'burden' on them, and a 'burden' on us. It can also set them up to become martyrs, and places the person with dementia into the role of being helpless. Some countries prefer to use the terms family carers, or caregivers. Some people use terms like enabler or supporter. We use the term BUB, or care partner.

It is however an important topic, and one that needs deeper exploration. If caring for people with dementia removes all of their basic rights and power, then it is not really care.

If the role of being a family carer or supporter allows care partners (family care partners or paid care partners) to blame us for how hard it is for them, it degrades us and, ultimately, their love for us.

In 2012 I nicknamed my husband BUB, or *Back-Up Brain,* and we find this terminology far easier to live with than carer or even care partner. Being called a carer has the potential to strip away the person's other roles. It also gives others the power over the person with dementia.

My husband says he cared for me long before I had dementia, and objects to this title or label. He is my best friend and husband, and sometimes he supports me. Sometimes I support him. That is what friends and couples do. Hence the term BUB. He is my best friend and my husband, and to start calling him my 'carer' simply denigrates us both.

If you think about how you use a back-up on your computer, the term BUB works the same way. You don't ask the back-up to do the tasks that the computer does, you only use it when the computer crashes, freezes or needs a reboot. We think of a Back-Up Brain as being the same as the hard drive in a computer. He said recently, it empowers him to be by my side and *with or alongside me,* rather than to *care for me,* a subtle but significant difference.

And so it is with my dear husband, who helps me live more fully with the symptoms of dementia. We have learned together to live with dementia, in ways that don't inhibit or restrict me as a person, and in ways that help to keep our love alive, way above the daily changes and traumas that can also be the *living with dementia.* He does not take away my dignity and power to do things for myself, but instead assists me from the sidelines, there when I ask for help; sometimes offering help if he sees me 'stumbling'.

Offering is also a key word here, as he does not enforce his opinions or help, but rather acts as my Back-Up Brain, my hard drive, the one that is fading, but with effort, and sometimes assistance, can still function well. It also empowers me to feel less of a failure, and less guilty about what is happening (failure, only in the sense of having to accept there are so many things I simply cannot do alone any more). I am the only one on this (my) train (person with dementia) who knows what is going on in my mind. Your imagination is far worse than anything you can actually tell, and your interpretation of what you think is best for me is simply that – your interpretation.

I read a lot and come across what was happening (to me) through textbooks and online articles and blogs. It is almost exclusively the words of those with dementia that really ring true for me. I'm sure it is the same for the people who love and live with us.

Most of the time at least for now, I don't often need my Back-Up Brain, but it is supportive to know it is there, and I need it more often as life goes on. Although it requires an enormous amount of effort on my part to function, I am happier doing this than relinquishing all of my responsibilities or abilities. Of course, many people discount this effort, thinking that there is nothing wrong with me; they don't see my endless notes and other coping mechanisms that I have developed to maintain my dignity and independence.

It would seem to me, if you want people to succumb to dementia quicker than they normally would, you should think for us, instead of letting us think for ourselves. If you want our brain to stop working then help us to stop using it.

But back to my term BUB and how it helps us. Peter says he find it stops him trying to take over and to know when to act and how. It sounds easy, but it's not; however, it does set some guidelines in the role each person has to play, and how to behave in and handle situations, and it does not strip me of my power nor give him all the control.

As a couple, we need to plan, without my husband trying to control my life too much – it is our struggle as a couple, but it is also my struggle, and my husband is there to support and advocate when I can't, not to live my life for me or, more importantly, to stop me living my own life. Dementia has changed the sense of 'us', in that he is now probably more important to me, sort of like being my lifeline. We don't know where we are heading but we are going there together.

Since I have been diagnosed with dementia, most of the things I have read have been written by people without dementia. Of course, family care partners also have significant reactions to the person they love having dementia, but becoming 'care partners' can give them all the power, and takes away ours. I continue to have deep concerns about how so many family care partners publicly write or speak out about how difficult this role is for them, and usually find it distressing, and it negatively and significantly impacts my shame, my deep sense of being a burden to my family and friends and my guilt.

CHAPTER 24

Care Partners Speaking Out Publicly About People with Dementia

To begin this section, I would like to acknowledge the amazing love, physical care and support that millions of family care partners provide for their loved ones. I have been a family care partner and legal guardian more than once, and know well of the emotional and physical drain, and how hard it is to self-care or take time out. I totally understand that. Friends like Charmaine and Beth in the UK, Michael in the USA, Lynda in Kiama, Sue in Brisbane, and many others I know personally or online, or the four beautiful women who started a support group called Tender Loving Carers in Adelaide, and many others I know in Australia and overseas have provided amazing support. Of course, this includes my husband. They are or were providing amazing support and love for those of us in their life who have or had dementia.

At no time do I ever wish to denigrate this amazing group of people – those mentioned here, and the millions of others supporting someone with dementia who they love.

Dementia is a unique illness, one that produces a need for the gradual increasing of physical care, but along the way starts to remove the previous relationships, those very things that created the bond in the first place.

What is it like for a partner, having accumulated years or decades of shared experiences, and huge networks of emotional connections between the couple, or the parent and adult child, when slowly, these relational fixtures are lost? I think that adds a huge layer of complexity, as the care partner is striving to sustain a relationship that is slowly evaporating, and won't end up existing at all. I have often read of adult children, commiserating on the fact their mum or dad is no longer able to be a parent, in the sense of a confidant or emotional support, and they are the ones having to switch roles. I know this to be difficult both emotionally and physically, through personal experience.

Unfortunately, in many cases, particularly those involving adult children caring for parents with dementia, or a partner caring for someone, a husband or wife, married, defacto or other, theirs is not the only relationship in jeopardy. The relationships you have with others tend to take a back seat, and your family and friends can drop away, simply because you don't have the time to see them as often, or they have disappeared due to the fear and stigma of the diagnosis of dementia. This can have an extremely deleterious effect on the health of the care partner, due to a lack of support, which I suppose is partly why so many write blogs or books about it, or speak out. The difficult and isolating role of being a care partner is hard work, and I am sure loneliness gets to them too.

However, I do feel I have a right, and that it is timely, for me to give my thoughts about the impact on people with dementia of those without dementia who speak or write publicly about a loved one with dementia.

Over the last year or so, there has been a lot more to be found online by people with dementia, but still the number of books and websites of, by and for care partners remains overwhelming. I have to say, I am unhappy about how often we (people with dementia) are referred to by care partners, researchers and professionals as burdens, or as challenging behaviours, and as sufferers, and how annoying and offensive it is to keep reading things like the comments below.

Some books and blogs are beautiful loving tributes to the person who has or had dementia, but many are also less than palatable, and simply increase my sense of guilt and shame. Care partners are no braver than people with dementia, and yet they often come out sounding like the heroes. We are all heroes, and for people with dementia, losing our own identity is terrifying, and painful. Having the insight it is happening, and knowing of the loss we are 'causing' those we love is hideous.

In a book on caring for his parents with dementia, a family care partner wrote things like:

> How to handle a crying spell at bed-time, or why she's suddenly become stubborn as a mule.

I wonder how this family care partner would feel if that was written about him or her? And 'she' has not suddenly become stubborn as a mule, she more likely was not able to communicate a need, or felt she was being forced to do something against her will. That is not being stubborn as a mule. That is the care partner not understanding her needs.

These types of conversations horrify and offend me, and if my husband wrote about me like that, I guarantee I would come back and haunt him. This person also wrote:

> When caring for someone who is suffering from Alzheimer's or dementia, be prepared to face hardships unlike anything you have encountered before.

If family care partners had any sense of respect for people with dementia, they would not be writing about the person, 'their loved one', in their family living with dementia, in this way.

The 'burden' this places on us is profound, and extremely emotionally disAbling and often offensive. We already feel profound guilt, and a burden on our family and friends, and society in general, and this makes that much worse. And we may be suffering some of the time, but many people with dementia have been asking for many years not to be labelled as *sufferers*, in the same way that no-one would call us retards. From my experience, the care partners are suffering far more than we are, as they have to watch us change and die. My husband, also my BUB or care partner, totally agrees with me on this one.

As difficult as this topic is, I first need to say I don't have any reluctance to acknowledge the challenges of caring for someone with dementia. I have been a family care partner, and understand it perfectly. However, it is a thorny thing for me to write about because I risk being too honest with my thoughts.

When I started feeling aggravated by some of the things family care partners were saying or writing publicly about caring for a loved one with dementia, I thought at first it was just me feeling annoyed that they spoke so loudly about the trauma of being a care partner, which very much worsens the guilt I feel; the guilt of being that burden! I fully accept and understand from personal experience that family care partners need support, but do wonder how they would feel if people with dementia all started speaking and writing publicly about how difficult their 'behaviours' can be or how mean or controlling they sometimes are or sound. I wonder if they would like to be publicly blamed for our 'behaviours of concern'.

Sometimes I wonder how they dare to publicly speak about a disease which they don't have. They can easily get support from their own groups, because they are not living with the disAbilities of dementia, and they could have their whinge or sharing about their guilt and loss of life outside of caring for us within these groups. I have no issue with that; it is the public forums I find troubling. They are not facing a slow lingering death with confusion or memory loss that potentially takes away our sense of identity, very often with the insight and awareness of it happening in front of our eyes.

Knowing you are the cause of changes to your partner's lifestyle can bring on the most wretched guilt; watching someone you love battling with and trying to accept the changes in you, and to your relationship, is gruelling, again causing further guilt, but does that give them the right to talk about how hard it is for them, in front of us, which it is if it is in a public forum? Personally, I don't think so.

As people with dementia develop a louder global voice, and start to speak out about their own realities, I hope this might help care partners to see that writing or speaking so negatively about us is hurtful. I'm sure they mean for it to be a loving tribute, but most often, it does not sound or read like that. I read a post on Facebook a few months ago, written by a care partner whose husband had passed away a few months before, that is was 'the anniversary of the 3rd [or 4th, 5th or 6th] month of getting her life back'. I cried for her husband.

To the family care partners out there writing books or blogs or Facebook posts about people with dementia, be prepared for people with dementia who previously rarely had the right of reply; we are now starting to speak up.

I used to think I needed to keep quiet about how offensive family care partners can sometimes be, and was worried about offending them, especially having been one as I do personally know the many challenges faced by being one.

But, I am tired of being disrespected and offended. They write about us, 'their loved ones', about how hard it is 'caring' for us, and seemingly don't think about whether their words might upset us. It certainly seems we are not *suffering* as much as they are. Personally, I have had enough of it, and I know many other people with dementia who feel the same.

Reading or listening to care partners' words, about their pain and how emotionally draining and physically tiring it is caring for someone with dementia, initially makes me want to empathise, but I struggle to because it is too painful for me to think that I may cause it. People with dementia never willingly wish to cause our loved ones suffering but it is obvious that many think we do. This outpouring simply exacerbates things like my guilt, shame and loneliness.

As Wayne Dyer says, no-one else is responsible for your or my reactions, even pain or suffering; people with dementia are not responsible for the way care partners feel either. It is their reaction and they must take responsibility for it, and stop blaming us. My husband has chosen not to blame me, nor to speak out publicly about how difficult it may sometimes be for him, because quite simply, he does not wish to offend me or make my own anguish worse. He always says it is not my fault I have dementia, and it is not me personally who is causing the symptoms and changes. He married me, he says, for better or worse, and just because

I have dementia, he feels, is not reason to start blaming me for it being worse.

Just like the language of dementia, if it is not okay to refer to me as retarded, then it is not okay to keep writing about how hard 'we' make it for family care partners. Many can make it harder for the person living with dementia, but do we keep yelling this out in public...no, we have more respect than that, or perhaps some people with dementia keep quiet because they are frightened love and support will be withdrawn if they do. I have seen this happen in residential aged care, where a resident or family member makes a complaint, and then some kind of punishment or a withdrawal of services take place. I have no doubts this would happen in the community and inside the privacy of homes. I've always been open enough to speak about some of the things that are less acceptable or less palatable, willing to cause a stir if needed, as creating change is more important to me than egos or others' opinions. Whether that means I am brave or stupid remains to be seen!

The learned helplessness, brought on initially by Prescribed Disengagement®, is simply exacerbated by this negative outpouring of their suffering, not ours. In fact, unlike the message they continue to give out, many of us are not suffering that much at all from dementia, in the sense of living 'devastating, horrific, and tragic' lives.

Giving up on trying to live beyond dementia is made easier by their outpouring. The loss of hope is exacerbated. It increases our already overwhelming and deep sense of guilt. It is already painful, with feelings of shame and humiliation, and the experience of stigma, discrimination and isolation, and I feel it would be helpful to us all if it stopped.

CHAPTER 25

Guilt

DEMENTIA AND ME[1]

What the hell happened to my brain
diagnosed with dementia when I was much too young
my children still at school
a deadly terminal disease affecting
memory, thinking, perception, judgment, language and
speech

But worse than that, affecting my
life, family, friendships, my sense of self, my identity
and a bucket load of guilt
truckloads of stigma discrimination and isolation
loss of dreams, and grief
sadness, disbelief, lost employment

And yet a new purpose of advocacy and activism
to bring about change
to stop the blatant abuse of the most basic of human rights
of people diagnosed with dementia, young or old
fewer old friends, new global friendships

The role of educator
teaching global lessons to academics and carers
hoping for and seeking change

---

1   http://kateswaffer.com/2014/09/20/dementia-and-me

searching for new ways for professionals
to discover we deserve the same as others with illness
not involuntary restraint

Eventually locked away in secure memory units
given drugs to make us compliant or physically restrained
the justification it's for our safety
helping aged care and hospitals comply with their duty of
    care
avoiding insurance claims

Worse than being locked in prison
the person with dementia
has not broken the law or done anything wrong
they are not criminals
they have a degenerative cognitive terminal disease
needing love and support

Support to remain engaged with pre-diagnosis activities
counselling to stay motivated
a disAbility access plan and assisted technologies
disAbility equipment, mentoring
positive psychology for our sense of wellbeing
and to be treated with dignity as whole human beings
Above all else.

(KATE SWAFFER 2014)

Being diagnosed with dementia brings with it a huge amount of guilt for both the person diagnosed, and their main care partner or supporter, and the reason I thought it worthwhile writing a short chapter about it is because so few ever acknowledge or talk about the guilt the person with dementia feels. I thought I'd begin by defining guilt.

Mr Google defines it like this:[2]

> guilt / gilt / noun: guilt
>
> The fact of having committed a specified or implied offense or crime.

The Oxford online dictionary[3] says:

> The fact of having committed a specified or implied offence or crime.
>
> A feeling of having committed wrong or failed in an obligation

The synonyms on the Oxford site are: culpability, guiltiness, blameworthiness, wrongdoing, wrong, wrongfulness, criminality, unlawfulness, misconduct, delinquency, sin, sinfulness, iniquity; responsibility, accountability, liability, answerability.

To set the scene for the rest of this chapter, I am sharing this blog, *Big Life, Small Suitcase*,[4] written on 7 August 2014.

> Kate Legge wrote a piece in The Australian, March 10–11 called '*How do you shrink a big life into a small suitcase?*' It was around the same time I had an article published in the Australian Journal of Dementia Care called '*Human rights in residential aged care: a consumer's perspective*'. The two articles look at aged care, mine telling some tales of woe, hers telling of the good experience she has had with her father. The positive stories are few and far between, and I've been wondering why. Perhaps because of her career [journalist], their experience has been better? After all, it would be rather stupid for an aged care provider to provide poor care if they thought it might get written about publicly.

2   www.google.com/search?q=definition+of+guilt&ie=utf-8&oe=utf-8
3   www.oxforddictionaries.com/definition/english/guilt
4   http://kateswaffer.com/2014/04/07/big-life-small-suitcase

So how do you pack a lifetime into a small suitcase? I was confronted with this when I packed a suitcase of personal and special belongings of my friend Michael who passed away last year, to take to the UK to his family. I found this incredibly difficult when selecting items from his 57 years to pack into a suitcase. His family had requested some things, but as we went through his home and belongings before the trip, and to empty the house for sale, we came across various other items we felt belonged with his family. As I lifted the small suitcase at the airport for weighing and loading for the trip, the fragility of life struck me, and the visual of an actual suitcase, full of a very big life was overwhelmingly sad.

When we packed up my father in law's home, and packed his life into a suitcase to enter aged care, it was confronting, and sad, and he hated it. Every single day, he said he felt locked in prison. Every single day I felt as if I had been his jailer. My mother in law died in her own home, and I suspect this is the greatest gift we ever gave her, as at the time we were able to support dad and nurse her at home. When she left their home, dad would not allow the funeral home staff to cover her face, and she headed off into the sunset, with the wind in her hair, from her own home. No need to pack her life into a small suitcase, and not once did she have to endure the feeling she had been locked in jail. I'm glad Kate Legge has been able to tell of a good and positive experience in aged care, but I do believe she is still in the minority.

Having been advocating in this sector for a few years now, I have made many friends and colleagues who are working really hard to improve things in aged and dementia care, and I applaud them. They are working against the odds; low wages, complicated funding bodies, state and Federal government changes, and the challenge of providing good food, interesting activities, staff who really care, and who have been appropriately educated, can speak English, as well as provide translator services for their clients who don't speak it, and so on. In my state, they pay staff at the Zoo to clean out the excrement in the animal cages more than they pay our paid care partners!

The guilt of being the care partner

The guilt and devastation and anger, and the grief and loss my father-in-law and two very close family friends, for whom I was also legal guardian, felt at having to leave their own homes was horrific. The guilt I felt not being able to care for them at home was horrific. It has not gone away.

After placing Dad and my young friend in a nursing home, both with different types of dementia, and both unable to live alone in their own homes, I was relieved that they were 'safe'. I was also riddled with guilt; I cried when I was home alone, wondering did we do the right thing. Every time we went to see them, they wanted me to take them home; it almost broke my heart. I feel like I took everything away from them. I'm not sure you ever get over this guilt.

My husband and I have talked many times about the guilt we feel for having placed his father into residential aged care, and in particular into high care for the last five months of his life. The term 'high care' is a bit of an anomaly, as most 'homes' generally do not offer care for the whole person. They do the basic tasks (for example, washing and dressing them, providing in many cases inedible food), but they do not treat their residents as if they are living in 'the last home of their life'. So to call it 'care' is in many sites really a misnomer. The residents are locked in, and feel like they are in prison. My father-in-law did. My young friend in aged care did. I know I would.

Our guilt is often tempered by the rational discussions we have about how even if my husband was retired and home full time, it would have been a gargantuan task. We now understand the great gift we gave my mother-in-law by nursing her at home, and allowing her to die in her own home.

The guilt of placing Dad and others I was legal guardian for into a residential aged care home still sits heavily, gently resting deep inside our hearts, never quite going away, gnawing away at us and casually suggesting we 'did something wrong'.

We know many loving partners of people with dementia who have had no choice than to move their loved ones into residential care, and most say they too feel this guilt, even though logically they did have no choice, and it was a decision made in the very best interest of their beloved one.

I want to say here that I personally understand that it is not possible for every person with dementia who 'wishes' to die at home to be able to die at home. In many cases the 'sole' family care partner or supporter can no longer care for them on at home. They just can't do it, and it would be wrong for them to try when they reach the point when they know they can't, or it is seriously affecting their own health.

The guilt of the person diagnosed with dementia

On the other hand, this topic or issue has not been researched or explored. In general, it is not thought about or acknowledged, but as one person diagnosed with dementia, I have felt guilty on an ongoing basis. No amount of rational thought takes it away. No amount of reassurance from my husband or friends dissolves it.

Every time, yes, every single time I have to ask someone to take me out in a car because I am no longer allowed to hold a licence to drive, I feel guilty. Everyone says they don't mind. I still feel guilty, and often put off going out because of it. It heightens the losses, and my dependence, and it reminds me I have dementia, so no chance of staying in the denial bubble either. No respite from dementia and no respite from guilt. When my husband gets upset or sad, I feel guilt; when I forget his name, I feel guilt. When I get my sons mixed up, or can't remember the name of a friend, I feel guilt.

I feel guilt asking for assistance with using a calculator, or converting a file to an image. I feel guilt not always remembering to switch off the gas burners, and have on many occasions left them on all day when I have been out. I have signs to help stop me from doing it, but they don't always work either. I feel more guilt when I forget to read or refer to them. I feel guilt when I forget to take my medication, even though there are multiple reminders. I've often wondered why this is, and I think is it because it means my husband has to remember more for me, be a more active Back-Up Brain. I feel guilt for rarely going to the movies with him any more, or going out to parties. Our life has changed, and it is all because I have a diagnosis of dementia, and the bloody symptoms get in the way of the life we had before. And dementia is not going away.

Oh, and that is on top of the shame, humiliation and embarrassment of not being able to remember or do things others can still do. When my parents used to visit from the country, and I could not offer to pick them up from the airport if they had flown in, I felt guilt.

Having dementia means I feel a burden, so to be talked about in the literature as a burden, and then publicly in blogs and books, and spoken about in presentations by care partners of how much their loved one with dementia was (is) a burden, even when I feel perhaps my feelings of guilt are fading, they come back with a vengeance. I regularly apologise to my husband for having dementia. He regularly tells me not to. I still feel guilt, and that I am a burden to him and others.

And then I need to talk about the ugly fear factor!

We fear of our future, of getting worse, which we are told will happen, and we see happening to many others we meet. Personally, we have had many people we know die from younger onset dementia in the last two years. Yes, we fear death too, but more than that, we fear being a bigger burden. Financially, emotionally, physically…a burden in every sense of the word, and our fear of worsening symptoms, which can only equate to more intense 'care' from someone, then we feel even more guilt.

Guilt is in fact wasted emotion, as you cannot change things that have happened, but that fact does not stop me from feeling it. I have chosen to get on with living in the best way possible, and work very hard to overcome the crippling effect of guilt, but it is a tough gig for sure. Being busy helps, my husband not speaking publicly about the 'burden' I have become helps, and even though he says I am not a 'burden' to him, I know our life has changed irrevocably, and it is because of dementia.

When I turn to tell my husband or sons, or a friend something, to share something with them, and suddenly cannot remember what I was about to say, or can no longer find the words, I feel guilt, as well as shame. There's often no-one there to take your thought, to take your frustration, to take your coffee, to take your hand.

When you share your moments and your life with someone, they permeate your very being. How you think, what you're thinking. When I cannot remember the restaurant we have been to, or the movie we watched on a plane, or what we had for dinner last night, or events from my children's lives, I feel sadness and guilt. Our conversations are emptier, because of my inability to recall parts of our life or understand things.

It is difficult and overwhelming because it's not just the loss of *my functions or capacity, it's the loss of our relationships, and lifestyle, and family stories. It's not one thing.* It's the daily, minute-by-minute reminders of this loss. *Every* moment *every* day I am reminded of this loss. I grieve *every day, and I feel guilt often, if not all of the time.* The reminders of these losses never go away.

The guilt and sadness can at times feel overwhelming, and there are days I am drowning under the weight of the losses of dementia, and the guilt. There are these constant reminders that have turned into continual good-byes to me and to my life, the one I had with my husband, sons, family and friends as we once we knew it. Of course I feel guilty.

CHAPTER 26

Who's Got the 'Challenging Behaviours'?

See the person, not the dementia.

(DEMENTIA ALLIANCE INTERNATIONAL 2014)

Managing Behavioural and Psychological Symptoms of Dementia (BPSD), 'challenging behaviours' or 'behaviours of concern' or managing the symptoms of dementia is a regular topic at conferences and forums about dementia, and one that drives me to a ranting distraction!

A recent study (Jeon *et al.* 2014) states the prevalence of Behavioural and Psychological Symptoms of Dementia (BPSD) in residential aged care (RAC) is high, occurring in over 78 per cent of people with dementia (13), and wandering is prevalent also, and it is obvious that wandering from a care setting unaccompanied may be dangerous. Perceptions of wandering by people without dementia is not always helpful to the provision of person-centred care on the issues of wandering (Kitwood 1997; Travers *et al.* 2015; Morhardt and Spira 2013; Sabat 2001); wandering versus walking is discussed here from the perspective of a person with dementia (Swaffer 2013):

I do a lot of walking around in circles, up and down the stairs to the bedroom, back to the office or kitchen, wondering why. If I was a resident in aged care, I would be labelled as wandering, rather than a person simply looking for something or going somewhere. The fact that I had forgotten what I was looking for or where I was going would not be written into the notes.

Algase *et al.* (2007) articulated this objective (they claim to be objective), empirically-founded definition to aid universal understanding of the behaviour:

> syndrome of dementia-related locomotion behavior having a frequent, repetitive, temporally-disordered and/or spatially disoriented nature that is manifested in lapping, random, and/or pacing patterns, some of which are associated with eloping, eloping attempts, or getting lost unless accompanied.

In *Behaviour Management – A Guide to Good Practice* (Burns *et al.* 2012, p.9) it states most behaviours are a form of communication. I remain confounded, however, that the overlying theme in this guide is around managing behaviour, rather than improving staff education on dementia and their client communication needs.

The term malignant social psychology coined by Kitwood (1997) and Kitwood and Bredin (1992) refers to the ways in which healthy others often unknowingly or innocently treat people with dementia in depersonalising ways that diminish their feelings of self-worth. Whilst the focus remains on challenging behaviours, rather than on attitudes and clinical practice, including care partners and registered or enrolled nurses and paid carers, it seems unlikely to me that person-centred care will ever be more than a tick box in documentation. I'm sure that the term BPSD negatively impacts that as well.

After attending a forum for nurses and other health professionals in clinical practice two years ago, more than half admitted to believing it appropriate to give people with dementia psychotropic drugs to 'manage behaviours'; I found this to be extremely distressing and worrying, in light of the fact they had all undertaken postgraduate up-skilling in dementia care.

Even though it is not considered best practice to do so, and even though *a diagnosis of dementia is the one contraindication of prescribing psychotropic drugs* – unless there is diagnosis of mental illness such as schizophrenia or bipolar disorder – many clinicians in the room of approximately 100 said it was still appropriate to do so.

As a consumer, I find it wrong there is a whole educational organisation devoted to managing 'challenging behaviours', with lists full of disrespectful words and terms, and whole chapters or sets of guidelines for how to manage them.

Before I was diagnosed with dementia, when I went walking, it was called walking, and even sometimes wandering, if I was simply walking to get some fresh air, or walking for exercise, or walking because I was bored, or walking to the shops, or walking for the sake of walking… now I would be labelled as a wanderer, and the ways to manage it would more likely be, according to many of the clinicians recently, with drugs.

People with dementia are not wanderers, absconders, screamers (yes, I heard that recently), poor feeders, feeders, aggressives, or 'not all there'…we are *people*, and sadly many caring for us have completely forgotten the ME in deMEntia.

Stated in an article by NPR.org, 'Old and overmedicated: the real drug problem in nursing homes':

Almost 300,000 nursing home residents are currently receiving antipsychotic drugs, usually to suppress the anxiety or aggression that can go with Alzheimer's disease and other dementia. (Jaffe 2014)

They go on to say:

Antipsychotics, however, are approved mainly to treat serious mental illnesses like schizophrenia and bipolar disorder. *When it comes to dementia patients, the drugs have a black box warning, saying that they can increase the risk for heart failure, infections and death.*

Professor Henry Brodaty and colleagues in their study, 'Halting Antipsychotic use in Long Term Care (HALT) Project',[1] propose a model for de-prescribing antipsychotics in residential care through person-centred approaches to managing challenging behaviours. A targeted, evidence-based training package has been developed to up-skill general practitioners and nursing home staff in this area, as well as in the quality use of medicines.

Bredesen's study (2014), mentioned in Chapter 28, may be significant to 'behaviours of concern' as if service providers and other health care professionals were to manage patients with dramatic lifestyle changes immediately after diagnosis, improvements may be more common. In this study patients had to avoid simple carbohydrates, gluten and processed foods, and they increased their fish intake, did yoga and meditated regularly. They were also instructed to take melatonin, get adequate sleep, incorporate vitamin B-12, vitamin D-3 and fish oil, and within six months, nine out of ten patients saw a noticeable improvement in memory. They are simple steps, and walking would easily be incorporated

---

1   www.dementiaresearch.org.au/index.php?option=com_dcrc&view=dcrc& layout=project&Itemid=142&pid=249

as a regular daily event for people with dementia and may also reduce what others see as problem behaviours including wandering, as well as other behaviours of concern like anxiety and poor sleep, as well as the physical benefits of regular exercise such as improving muscle tone, strength and balance and reducing falls. Improving lifestyle factors also improve wellbeing and quality of life, and introducing them in the early stages of the disease may also significantly reduce the need for residential care.

The other learning from the BPSD guidelines is they recommend behaviour charting as a useful tool to confirm the information from the initial referral. They claim charting behaviour over several days will provide accurate, objective information and a baseline measure of the behaviour. Three days is typically suggested for most BPSD; however, two sessions of 24 hours each with a break in between is recommended for wandering behaviours. I believe if we actually provide person-centred care, and move away from this methodology, most 'behaviours of concern' would never surface.

Finally, at least for now on this topic, I remain extremely sceptical about the use of the term Behavioural and Psychological Symptoms of Dementia (BPSD) and believe the categorisation of behaviours into things like wandering, aggressive, absconder, screamer, poor feeders, and so on, simply increases the likelihood of person-centred care not being delivered, and of the stigma and discrimination continuing. It also ensures many in care remain locked up, 'for their own safety', even though it is more likely because of the lack of staff to properly care for people's needs as whole human beings.

It stops others seeing the whole person, instead focusing on a person's behaviour, not even a symptom of dementia, or a communication problem.

The official category BPSD was the result of a consensus conference in Lansdowne in 1996, and interestingly was sponsored by Janssen Pharmaceuticals, and it had a major impact on research, intervention, and definition of dementia. In terms of interventions, previously existing drugs, like the cognitive enhancers, began to be tested for non-cognitive outcomes such as activities of daily living, behaviour, and global outcome (Leibing 2014).

It appears from this article that the term BPSD has been developed by pharmaceutical companies, and my increasingly cynical consumer/student perspective suggests to me it was simply a way to define people with dementia in ways that can be managed by drugs, for example anti-anxiety or anti-agitation medications. People with dementia have been labelled disparagingly, to allow the prescribing of 'behaviour'-modifying drugs, simply because of a failure of the pharmaceutical industry to find enough dementia (disease) modifying drugs or drugs for a cure. They have to sell something after all…

I think, sadly, there are books and complete guides and whole chapters on managing challenging behaviours, and these can surely only support and exacerbate stigma and poor care. My major research project for 2016 and perhaps beyond is to review all of the research articles, books, guides and guidelines, and see if there might be a better way forward, that properly honours the person with dementia and their right to good care that is person- and relationship-centred, but that also does not infringe on their human rights. Better care, surely, will ultimately cost the sector less, and yet it is not just a quick fix. The current approach ensures the low level of staffing found in most aged care homes is not easily noticed. With residents all drugged up to compliance, many barely able to speak, let alone get up and walk…or is that wander…that is the easy option.

Each week I am alerted to a new method of care, aimed at improving the lives and care of people with dementia. Until funding and staff levels change, I fail to see how most of them can have much of an impact. Tom Kitwood's person-centred care, written about many years ago, is still not in action at many of the aged care homes I have been in, and whilst we are always written up as a challenging behaviour, and spoken about that way by the whole sector, that may never change.

There is a whole book in me on this topic. Personally, I think the people who need managing most often are the staff who have people with dementia in their care…perhaps this will be the topic of a PhD.

I'd like to add one comment about walking. Walking is found to be an effective rehabilitation intervention, resulting in a significant improvement in mobility performance and improvement in balance (Sinclair, Morley and Vellas 2012). Walking not only enhances mobility, which is important as it affects not only ability to walk and move around, but also influences other areas such as eating, toileting, personal hygiene, and leisure activities (Squires and Hastings 2002). What on earth is the rationale or value of care providers stopping people with dementia from 'wandering'?

For now, I will leave this for another time and after more research, but I have added below a poem. I have written a few versions of the poem 'Wandering along the beach,' and many who have read it say it should be mandatory reading for those caring for a person with dementia. Many have also asked permission to print it and take to support meetings, or their workplace, as also happened with my list of '20 ways to more positively support a person with dementia'.[2] Feel free to go to my website and print it off for use in your own workplaces or homes.

WANDERING ALONG THE BEACH[3]

Before a diagnosis of dementia, if I went walking,
Even if I was 'wandering' through a shopping centre for
    pleasure,
It was still referred to as walking
Wandering along the beach with the sand between my toes
Was still considered walking
When I go walking, even if I get lost, I am not a
    wanderer…
I am a person
Sometimes people like to go for walks
Even people with dementia
Sometimes people get lost
Even people without dementia
Sometimes people walk because they are looking for
    something
Even people with dementia
Sometimes people go walking because they are bored
Even people with dementia
Sometimes people go walking because they might be trying
    to 'escape'
Or 'manage' the boredom of living in an aged care facility
They might be feeling like they are in prison…
Locked up even when they are not criminals…
Sometimes people walk for exercise

---

2   http://kateswaffer.com/2014/06/05/20-things-not-to-say-or-do-to-a-person-with-dementia

3   http://kateswaffer.com/2014/11/29/wandering-along-the-beach

Even people with dementia
Before aged care, people were involved in habitual walking
   almost all the time...
Walking to the kitchen to get a cup of tea,
Walking to the bathroom,
Walking to the shed,
Walking to the clothesline,
Walking to the shops...
Living in aged care does not mean people with dementia
   wish to stop walking
Oddly, before a diagnosis dementia, doctors tell us to get or
   keep fit,
And that walking is one of the best exercises for us...
Even more oddly, when we have dementia this must stop
Walking is then referred to as wandering
A challenging behaviour that needs managing
People with dementia are still 'real' people
Living their lives just as they did before acquiring the label
   of dementia
People with dementia are not wanderers,
Nor poor feeders, aggressives, or demented sufferers
People with dementia still wish to live well
But get very little support from others for well-being
Or for improving our quality of life
Including for walking
Walking is good for us and fun...
It is not a challenging behaviour.

CHAPTER 27

Dementia and Common Sense

I often think about common sense, and wonder if it has gone these days – not just in dementia care, but almost everywhere. Perhaps it's the farm girl coming out in me, but I think common sense is becoming a lost art, and one we should work on retrieving, especially in dementia care.

The desire and intent to improve and provide better care for people with dementia seems high in the sector, especially amongst service providers and researchers, and for that, I am truly delighted. However, whilst we do need evidence-based practice, we also need some good old-fashioned common sense in our core plans. This definitely seems to be missing. We have all this 'education' and evidence-based research to inform us, but very little common sense being used in dementia care. Here are a few examples.

We all know the positive effects of sunlight on mood, and the health issues such as vitamin D deficiency, and then we wonder why people living in residential care become unhappy, and why their symptoms of dementia get worse. Surely it is logical that never going outside into the sunshine will lower mood and happiness, and reduce the vitamin D in our bodies, both potentially negatively effecting dementia symptoms.

We all know the positive effects of daily exercise, but, mostly, people in residential aged care are lucky to get any exercise at all, other than walking to the bathroom or the dining room, and that is often with help to save time. We know the negative effects on our physical and emotional health, including falls risk, when we don't exercise. This therefore also negatively affects people with dementia.

We all know the positive effects of healthy, nourishing food, made from fresh produce, served to us in a way that look appetising and appealing, and smells and *tastes* good. We also know how we would feel if we were made to eat food that was boring, mushy or that we disliked. Not wanting to eat the food served up also affects the person and their dementia.

We all like to feel we have control, and that having some control of our own life increases many things, such as our positive outlook and self-esteem. Yet, all control is taken away from people living in residential care. This is in spite of the fact that residential aged care is beautifully marketed as 'your new home'. Really, your new home, and you can't get out (no, you are not given a key), and you have almost no say in how you live, when and what you eat, the music you listen to, or the activities available to you. People with dementia are already losing control of their functioning, their capacity, their abilities, so to take even more control away from them when they go into residential care can only make them sad, unhappy, anxious and yes, even angry. This additional lost control might also have something to do with some of the 'behaviours of concern' many people are being physically or chemically restrained for.

We all know the positive effects of meaningful activities, of engaging in the hobbies and activities we enjoy, such as gardening or music. Yet I often see activity rooms in residential care and 'day' respite, full of people looking bored, playing bingo or doing other meaningless group activities. This allows for fewer members of staff, and less work in planning, but is not person centred in any way.

We all know the positive effects of normal socialising and going out to community events, yet rarely do I ever hear of people in residential care being taken out to events like concerts. Instead, we bring activities in-house to the residents, all sitting around the 'day room' or 'activity room'. Surely it would be far more fun going *out* to the theatre or the movies, and not doing so negatively affects people with dementia as well.

We know that many of the family and friends drop away when someone is diagnosed with dementia, and then, when they move into residential care, visitors dwindle even more. Research clearly support this. So, supporting people who live in residential care homes to socialise in normal ways has to be good for them in ways other than it being person centred. Improving mood, happiness and wellbeing, perceived or otherwise, as well as giving them back some sense of control has to be a good thing, surely?

We know that for all other disease or illnesses, changing lifestyle factors improves our chances of recovery or reducing the impact of the illness. Increasing exercise, rehabilitation, improving nutrition, getting sunlight, and working our brains hard are all positive interventions that improve our wellbeing, even if they are not a cure.

It makes good common sense to provide care for people with dementia that provides the same support as any other disease. Who knows, if they start to feel happier simply due to increased serotonin from exercising, and have less falls because of some regular resistance and balance exercises, it might actually be good for them, and even slow down the deterioration caused by dementia. It might even reduce their 'challenging behaviours'.

Let's bring back some good old-fashioned common sense, especially in the dementia care sector.

————————————————————

CHAPTER 28

Interventions for Dementia

Some time ago, I wrote *'dementia is awkward to live with'*. The thing that stands out in that phrase for me now is 'to live with', as I suspect this is a significant key to remaining positive. When first diagnosed, I was told to 'give up work, give up study, and start living for the time I had left', which is unhelpful, unethical and unhealthy, and which I termed Prescribed Disengagement®.

If I had taken this advice and stopped living a meaningful and engaged life, that had real value, I often wonder would the symptoms of dementia have sped up, would my experience have been less positive, or would my ability to still achieve things that have true meaning to my existence have slowed down or come to a halt. Of course, this is only something I can speculate on, but I *believe* this would have happened.

Dr Bruce Lipton, in his book, *The Biology of Belief* (2011), supports the role of belief as a factor in our ability to change health outcomes. In an overview about the book on his website, it says:

> The implications of this research radically change our understanding of life. It shows that genes and DNA do not control our biology; that instead DNA is controlled

by signals from outside the cell, including the energetic messages emanating from our positive and negative thoughts. Dr Lipton's profoundly hopeful synthesis of the latest and best research in cell biology and quantum physics is being hailed as a major breakthrough showing that our bodies can be changed as we retrain our thinking.

I constantly review and work on retraining my thinking, in the belief I can change my cells. I continue to work on a neuroplasticity exercise programme, in the belief I will create new pathways in my brain. Some say this is wishful thinking. I simply say, why not try these things, and to some extent they do seem to be working for me. Even so, the last few weeks, I have been finding the symptoms of dementia have been changing, and my paddling has needed to be a lot harder to keep afloat.

In the process of the struggle, I've often given myself a hard time, and spend too much time focusing on my deficits, rather than what I can still do, the very thing I ask people caring for someone with dementia not to do! So tomorrow, I might write about what it is I can still do, and then get on with doing it!

Dementia is still awkward to live with, but living beyond dementia for as long as I possibly can with the assets I still have is what I must do. I've always believed 'good things come to those who work their asses off and never give up!' The next section explains how I do that. Organisations like Alzheimer's Australia are also now supporting brain health as prevention, with their site 'Your Brain Matters – a guide to healthy hearts and minds'.[1] But this is not enough, and globally we need so much more than is currently being offered post-diagnosis.

---

1   http://fightdementia.org.au/about-dementia-and-memory-loss/am-i-at-risk/your-brain-matters

Non-pharmacological and positive psychosocial interventions

A non-pharmacological intervention is any intervention such as exercise or physical rehabilitation that does not involve drugs; it refers to therapy that does not involve drugs. A psychosocial intervention is a broad term used to describe different ways to support people to overcome challenges and maintain good mental health, and they also do not involve the use of medication.

Possibly for the first time a study has shown definitively that environmental factors are crucial in preventing dementia. Late last year British health charity Age UK reviewed academic studies and data and found that 76 per cent of cognitive decline is down to lifestyle, including factors like level of education. The report, called *The Disconnected Mind*, has led to five steps being suggested to help prevent the development of dementia conditions, such as Alzheimer's disease.

Regular physical exercise is the most important factor, as well as a healthy diet, not smoking and drinking in moderation. Avoiding or treating diabetes, high blood pressure and obesity is also crucial.

A study of British people conducted over 30 years found that men aged between 45 and 59 who ticked four or five of those lifestyle boxes had a 36 per cent lower chance of developing dementia than those who did not.

> *While there's still no cure or way to reverse dementia, this evidence shows that there are simple and effective ways to reduce our risk of developing it to begin with.* This development comes hot on the heels of the discovery of the brain's weak spot that allows the development of dementia, so the armoury for fighting cognitive decline seems to be ever increasing.
>
> (Caroline Abrahams, Age UK)

Read more about The Disconnected Mind research project that aims to discover how our thinking skills change with age, and what we can do to protect our cognitive health in later life, funded by Age UK.[2]

Dale Bredesen (2014) has done a study 'Reversal of cognitive decline: a novel therapeutic program' at the University of California in Los Angeles. Ten memory-loss patients, some with brain-scan-confirmed patterns of Alzheimer's, participated in a small trial called Metabolic Enhancement for Neuro Degeneration (MEND). Nine of the ten displayed subjective or objective improvement in cognition beginning within three to six months, the only failure to improve being a patient with very late stage Alzheimer's disease.

Six of the patients had previously stopped working or were struggling with their jobs at the time of presentation, and all were able to return to work or continue working with improved performance. Improvements have been sustained, and currently the longest patient follow-up is two and a half years from initial treatment, with sustained and noticeable improvement. These results suggest that a larger, more extensive trial of this therapeutic programme is warranted. The results also suggest that, at least early in the course, cognitive decline may be driven in large part by metabolic processes.

Improving wellbeing and quality of life in dementia

Non-pharmacological interventions, such as holistic options, improved diet, psychological and psychosocial interventions, have the potential to improve cognitive function and therefore improve the quality of life. They can

----

2   www.ageuk.org.uk/about-us/what-we-do/the-disconnected-mind

also delay institutionalisation, as well as reduce care partner strain and psychological illness, thereby increasing wellness, and perceived longevity. Minimal attention has been paid to the specific needs of people with dementia and their family members in the early stages of the disease. In the USA, there was a needs assessment carried out and participants expressed the need for practical information, financial and legal counselling, emotional support, and an interest in research, including clinical trials for the disease.

Little research had been done on the value of neurophysiotherapy, but evidence is slowly growing to support its benefits. Evidence to support the benefits of neuroplasticity and its ability to create new pathways in the brain is growing, and Norman Doidge (2012) cites examples of healing based purely on neuroplasticity training. Dr Bruce Lipton, in *The Biology of Belief* (2005, 2011) discusses Trans-cranial Magnetic Stimulation, used to treat depression and to improve cognition. He also discusses using the brain, and that the brain controls the behaviour of the body's cells. He states 'the overuse of prescription drugs provides a vacation from personal responsibility'. Dr Ross Walker (medical cardiologist) in his latest book *The Five Stages of Health* (2012) discusses how to cut through the mixed messages we get in the media about maintaining our health.

Happiness, peace and love are far more important to your overall health than the purely medical or physical things, and have more to do with wellness than we might think. Three of the stages discuss more than medical health; stage two (2) discusses Environmental Health, stage four (4) Emotional Health and stage five (5) discusses Mind Health, highlighting non-pharmacological interventions including the use of supplements, and the real value of things such as the cleansing of energies flowing through our bodies (our Chakras). He cites a study showing MRI proof of a reduction of Alzheimer's disease after a 12-month course of therapy. There is a body of clinical evidence slowly growing to support non-pharmacological interventions, by respected medical doctors, neurophysiotherapists and scientists. The South Australian government funded Dr Martin Seligman, a prominent psychologist, as one of their Thinkers In Residence in 2012; he not only supports the notion of wellness based on positive psychology and lifestyle options, he travels the world promoting it.

Norman Doidge's book, *The Brain that Changes Itself,* anecdotally supports brain plasticity and its role in changing the pathways in our brain to improve function, and his second book on neuroplasticity, *The Brain's Way of Healing,* proves it with solid evidence. If you haven't read these books, make an effort to do so, even if you need someone to read them to you due to changes in visual abilities.

Based on my own experience, I believe if the medical community and service providers of dementia and dementia care don't start to embrace these interventions soon, not only are they doing their clients a grave disservice, the lost opportunities in the early stages of dementia, when we have a better chance of these types of interventions making a difference, will increase the economic impact of dementia worldwide.

Interestingly, even non-religious people will believe in a 'God miracle' if a patient is cured, and yet so few in the medical arena are willing to believe in patients who have either cured themselves, or improved their outcomes using non-pharmacological or positive psychological interventions.

The use of pharmacological interventions for dementia, which are not a cure, but may slow down the progression, excludes a minimum of 50 per cent of everyone diagnosed with dementia, and until very recently, researchers, service providers and the medical community have offered *nothing* to those of us where medication is not available. Thankfully, the tide is turning and a few are now supporting us to proactively care for ourselves.

Neuroplasticity exercises, transcendental meditation, self-hypnosis, improved diet, supplements, exercise, tertiary education, volunteering, counselling, creative writing, poetry, music therapy and laughter have ensured I have reached wellbeing through engagement, fun and meaning. Resilience has also been vital to remaining positive. A phenomenological approach to this illness is my other key to positivity.

If it was a stroke that gave me cognitive impairment aged 49, I would have been authentically rehabilitated in a brain injury unit, and if possible, sent back to work. It was very concerning to read during my Master's degree the book *Perspectives on Rehabilitation and Dementia* (Marshall 2005) which was born from a conference on the importance of rehabilitation and dementia nine years ago, and then to be communicating with students on the university discussion board, who were also registered nurses working in rehabilitation units, and who see dementia and aged care patients, but who admitted to never having considered rehabilitation interventions for these patients. It concerns me deeply that we are not being offered the same level of care as any other disease group. This 'pathway to dying' rather than the 'pathway to living as well as possible' is still the norm, and needs to change.

Rehabilitation is valuable and worthwhile for the elderly and for people with dementia, regardless of the amount of evidence-based research to support it. Quite simply, there are times in caring for people with dementia that research needs to come second to quality of life and common sense, including simple things like joy and perceived wellbeing.

The whole of health is impacted by physical activity, and walking is the one exercise that costs nothing, other than time. Intent and good will is required by aged care providers, however the benefits in terms of improved outcomes for residents would be significant. Not only will other more expensive interventions be reduced, having mobile clients who can manage their own daily needs would be beneficial to all, including costs savings to management.

The non-pharmacological and positive psychosocial interventions for dementia that I use

The self-prescribed interventions, now supported by my neurophysiotherapist, fill up a lot of my days, and I consider them the 'Olympics training of my life'. So far, they seem to be working:

- advocacy and activism

- public speaking

- studying

- phenomenology

- autoethnography

- neuroplasticity brain and body training

- neurophysiotherapy

- exercise six days/week – walking, balance exercises and stretching

- Authentic Brain Injury Rehabilitation
- hydrotherapy
- Pilates
- speech pathology (why is this not in care plans for people with dementia? We all have speech, word-finding or language impairment)
- occupational therapy
- blogging
- creative writing
- poetry
- healthy nutrition – especially avoiding processed sugar
- supplements
- music
- Mind Mapping
- volunteering
- laughter and a lot of humour
- exploring my spiritual life
- love
- reading
- belief
- Transcendental Meditation, 20 minutes, three times a day
- self-hypnosis for pain relief to prevent negative cognitive effects of medication

- mindfulness

- family time with my husband and sons

- nurturing friendships

- social media

- working on my personal resilience

- living every day as if it is my last, just in case it is.

Other interventions could include things like art, singing in a choir, dancing, fishing, or any other usual recreational or social activity. Living your life in the same way you did before diagnosis is, perhaps, the best intervention for dementia of all, if that is what you want to do! The one thing I would definitely be displaying a 'challenging behaviour' over would be if you made me play bingo!

A phenomenological approach to this illness has been a significant key to my positivity; that is, studying the nature of things as they are, and investigating and describing my conscious experience in all its varieties without reference to the question of whether what is experienced is objectively real. My blogging has allowed me to do this, not only by pushing me to think about it, but to try to express it in a way that has clarity and is meaningful for others to share or to learn from. Treating my symptoms as the gateway to supporting disAbilities rather than managing them as if I am dying, and managing emotional changes with grief counselling and positive engagement, rather than treating symptoms with drugs, have become paramount to my wellbeing and perceived longevity.

If I had been referred to the brain injury unit (in the early stages, dementia is not that different), I would have been proactively *treated* to live the very best life possible with the *injury* I have. Suggesting I disengage from my meaningful life, and take up activities other people thought might sustain my soul, was not only illogical, it was insulting and unethical. Initially it seemed I should join in, I should be grateful for the services people are trying so hard to provide, often with limited funding and resources. But I have found mostly I get no enjoyment from engaging in things that I am not interested in (doh!).

Often I still wonder, are most of the medical profession and service providers not more actively looking for ways to improve our lives in truly meaningful ways, as well as enhancing our perceptions of longevity, rather than simply planning for our demise? Please don't simply shut us away in the activities rooms, doing things others perceive we might enjoy or get meaning from. Ask us what we want, who we used to be, and then work collaboratively with us rather than for us, in an effort to allow us to continue with our lives in productive and meaningful ways. And always, in the same way as we would be told with cardiac disease or diabetes, promote looking after our health.

Professor Steve Iliffe, Professor of Primary Care for Older People, Research Department of Primary Care and Population Health, University College London, was one of the keynote presenters at the New Zealand Alzheimer's Biennial conference[3] in 2013, presenting on *Prevention, health promotion and early intervention in dementia.* I also presented at this conference a number of times, and you can see an interview[4] I gave on the Paul Henry Show if you are really keen! Anyway back to Steve… He discussed what he thought about my view of treating the symptoms of dementia as disAbilities, or seeing dementia as a disease, and decided

---

3   www.alzheimers.org.nz/getmedia/c4ab5ff3-aa30-46f9-8969-ed0c956efcfd/
     Prof_Steve_Iliffe.pdf.aspx
4   www.3news.co.nz/tvshows/paulhenryshow/when-dementia-hits-2014
     111223#axzz3oMk6jFuP

my view of treating it as a disAbility was preferable when thinking about better managing outcomes for patients. He believes Primary Prevention must help patients reduce heart disease statins, control blood pressure, prevent diabetes, help patients to stop smoking, increase habitual exercise, and reduce poverty through education. He commented with some cynicism that before a diagnosis of dementia, doctors tell their patients to exercise, and that walking is one of the best exercises, and after a diagnosis of dementia, they must stop walking (wandering), and of course, that resonated with me! These factors all link in with healthy lifestyle and many of the non-pharmacological interventions for dementia. In his summary, he stated 1) dementia prevention is already underway (under other names), 2) preventative activities (and beneficial social trends) may already be working, 3) obesity and diabetes will challenge prevention plans, and 4) that downstream interventions need more research, but there are already promising interventions.

There is probably another book in me to further elucidate non-pharmacological and positive psychosocial interventions, and their value, but that is for another day. Dr Shibley Rahman's two books *Living Well with Dementia: The Importance of the Person and the Environment for Wellbeing* (2014), and *Living Better with Dementia: Good Practice and Innovation for the Future* (2015), both go into a lot of detail on living beyond dementia, and Shibley is, in my very humble opinion, correctly going against the current trend of medicalisation of dementia that continues, in an effort to better support people with dementia to live beyond dementia, their care partners to be well-informed, and for health care providers, doctors and clinicians included, to be more concerned with personhood and wellbeing for people with dementia, and to see us as whole people. And thank goodness!

CHAPTER 29

Blogging and Writing as Interventions for Dementia

A BRAVE NEW WORLD

Geeks, nerds, bloggers and me
Plugins widgets tags akismets
A new world to marvel
Inspire, educate and engage
Speakers to cover all bases
Sunshine dancing and beer
Ripples of new dreams
Masses of motivation
This brave new world
Creating memories
Retaining memories
Blogging works for me

(KATE SWAFFER 2011)

Blogging feels like it is an autobiography in progress, and having an active blog, and a few Twitter and Facebook followers or friends, very much feels like I have a whole group of narrative therapists, as well as a fabulous bunch of 'new friends', or pen pals. Blogging and writing have opened up my world and my heart, and definitely allowed me to be more discerning and to love myself more. Blogging, writing and poetry also feel like positive psychosocial interventions, as well as non-pharmacological interventions for dementia. It is hard work writing and editing, and I specifically choose writing poetry, and soon will have two new books published locally, one a complete book of haikus; I specifically choose to write haikus because that form of poetry makes my brain work harder.

The art of handwriting and letter writing is becoming obsolete as we are all using text messaging, email, Twitter, Facebook and other types of social media. I have gathered lots of global friends via my blog, and now consider them to be pen pals, and am excited to be meeting a few of them soon when I travel to the UK. As a child, I had pen pals, and we wrote to each other for years, perhaps why I enjoy 'talking' to my blogging friends in the same way!

Wikipedia defines pen pals as 'people who regularly write to each other, particularly via postal mail'. It says:

> A penpal relationship is often used to practice reading and writing in a foreign language, to improve literacy, to learn more about other countries and life-styles, and to make friendships. As with any friendships in life, some people remain penpals for only a short time, while others continue to exchange letters and presents for life. Some penpals eventually arrange to meet face to face; sometimes leading to serious relationships.

Whilst the definition given above says postal mail is the most used, I believe internet communication has taken over, which is helpful to me, even though I prefer handwritten letters. I've spent the last couple of months in a rehabilitation unit, referred there by my neurologist to assist with the deficits of dementia. I am having trouble writing due to the acquired dyslexia, and have almost completely reverted to using the computer. The occupational therapist advised me to practise handwriting every day in an effort to see if I can improve it, or at least delay the impairment. I'm not sure it is working, but will keep practising in the same way I work on the other deficits.

As the world changes around us, we all must eventually accommodate the changes. My grandfather disliked change intensely, and when daylight saving came in, he refused to change his wrist watch, which almost drove Nan mad! I cannot imagine how he would cope with today's fast-paced changes, and suspect he would continue to post his beautiful handwritten letters. I loved and still love receiving handwritten cards and letters, and still write the occasional one, which I am told by the recipients they really love receiving.

Believe it or not, my blog is full of many wonderful pen pals, and some of my readers have told me they even print off each one to keep in case I shut down the blog. How lovely is that! Some people, of course, probably hate what I write, and on occasion have told me so. That's okay too; I don't like everything I read either, although if I don't like it, I usually just stop reading it, rather than writing to the author to tell them how awful their words are.

One of my gurus or mentors the late Dr Wayne Dyer, who I had the great pleasure and privilege of meeting in Adelaide once. He would not have remembered me, but I really hope I will always remember him. After David died through suicide, Wayne's books and motivational tapes helped me survive, helped me heal and helped me turn what was a tragedy and could have turned my life into a negative spiral of grief into something worthwhile and positive. His words helped me see through the sadness, to see the light in the darkness.

One of the things he did was send fan mail to those people who had written to him telling him how much they hated his writings, and then he sent the hate letters to his loving fans. It did, I am now sure, keep him and them very grounded. Even in a landslide election win, is it rarely more than 50 per cent of people who have voted for you, although when you start blogging, if you have not been a public person, you expect everyone will either love you or shut up! That is definitely not the case, and I now have a lot more respect for writers who have daily newspaper columns or who are in other public spaces.

Blogging has helped to bring back the dreaming, and to fill up the 'empty shell'. However, I have felt fear about blogging as I've been reminded that blogging is out there for the world to see, and might be fraught with danger. Danger of personal security, danger of people who dispute your ideas or don't like your creative work, and in my particular case, the risk of people who don't believe I have dementia because I choose to publicly share that part of my journey, using ways that are more commonly found to be deficit in people with dementia. It has been suggested that because I blog so openly about it, I have a responsibility to prove my authenticity, or at least that there may be people out there who won't believe me until I do.

I felt rather traumatised by the reminder of this. Increasing the fear factor is the people who know me, who are saying they don't believe I have dementia; people who have not spoken to me, but instead talk about their doubts behind my back. I have been helped to understand this was not meant maliciously or done with intent to slander, but it remains hurtful rather than helpful. This behaviour, whilst it may be meant with good intentions, merely intensifies my fear factor and undermines my ability to positively live with this pesky disease. It also greatly upsets my family, who live with this anxiety too.

Blogging...a living funeral

In one of my favourite books, *Tuesdays with Morrie*, Mitch Albom tells the true story of Morrie Schwartz who is dying of amyotrophic lateral sclerosis (ALS), also referred to as Lou Gehrig's disease, which is a form of motor neurone disease. A brave man with a positive view of life, Morrie believes one cannot learn how to live unless one knows how to die. Albom, an average journalist, tells this story about his favourite college professor who is dying and who changed his life by showing him reasons for existence, and the things we should cherish. He travels many miles and meets with Morrie on Tuesdays, and Mitch realises how much better his life is with all the time he spends with Morrie, and ultimately becomes a much better person. In this story, Mitch shares how Morrie has a *funeral* before he dies, so he can get to hear the things people say about him, which in turn offers him the opportunity to respond, to share his own love and answer any questions about his life his loved ones might ask. So often I have been to a funeral and found out so many things about someone whom I thought I knew, as well as having an overflowing basket full of questions that will remain unanswered forever. Morrie's *gift* to his family and friends is profound, and makes his death so much more meaningful.

Apart from becoming my memory bank, blogging has become my journal. It is the 21st-century diary, except that my blog readers get to read it before I die! How cool is that?! Well, it is for me anyway. Rather than having to wait until I die, they can share my thoughts, and see into my heart and soul. I have decided it definitely allows them, and me, to share more honestly and openly. Rather than have someone find my journals and diaries some time after death, and interpret them in ways that may not be authentic to who I am or what I meant (perhaps even publish them, without my permission), they are there, for all to read. They are there as a matter of public record, for anyone to respond to, to ask questions about if they can be bothered, or to ignore if they so choose. This *public blogging thing* has had a profound effect on me; it has opened me up to a world of new online friends, it has strengthened my relationships with those friends who are joining me on this ride, and has given me a new type of power over my own destiny. It may not be a living funeral, but it is an online version of that same deep intimacy and shared love.

Blogging and writing helps me find inner strength

The telling of clients' stories is an important component of the therapeutic process; whatever approach we use, our story will be a part of what we work with, so a sophisticated questioning of what stories or narratives are will benefit us. Narrative Therapy places people's accounts of their lives and relationships at the heart of the therapeutic process, and its main premise is that the telling and re-telling of experience by means of guided questioning can facilitate changed, more realistic perspectives, and open up possibilities for the person seeking assistance to position him- or herself more helpfully in relation to the issues brought to therapy (Mascher 2002; Payne 2006; Polkinghorne 2000; White, Morgan and Dulwich Centre 2006). The writing of narrative, either journaling, blogging, poetry or even sending letters can be something we can do on our own or with support, and the sharing stories offers us the experience of a 'therapist', that is, our family and friends. In the context of dementia, life stories and poetry writing, based around narrative of one's life, is not only valuable for us now, but has the potential to provide a detailed life history if we go into residential care.

There is some evidence to say poetry and other writing can help with emotional stability for family care partners (Anonymous 2009; Burack-Weiss and Ebrary 2006; Hagens, Beaman and Ryan 2003; Kidd 2009; Kidd, Zauszniewski and Morris 2011; Zeilig 2014) and it seems reasonable it may be therapeutic for a person with dementia. In my own personal experience of living with younger onset dementia, I believe writing poetry and blogging or writing about my life stories has been the key to keeping away the 'black dog' of depression and apathy, something so many with dementia experience. Writing about one's own experience allows exploration of support that promotes not only humanity and self-evaluation, but intimate sharing.

The expression of our lived experience of living with dementia, through writing life stories and poetry, allows us to explore our own behaviour in a non-threatening way, and for me has been extremely positive in my life. I seriously recommend it for others, not meaning it has to be a public blog like mine, but a regular exploration through writing – stories in a journal book, a private or public blog, poetry or narrative therapy – is a very effective way to not only catalogue your slowly disappearing world, but to make sense of it.

Finding the strength to overcome challenges is always the greatest challenge. For many, fear is the greatest challenge that holds us back from moving forward. Blogging and other writing has helped me overcome many of my fears.

Blogging helped me overcome my fear of writing and being published. Blogging and other writing have helped me overcome my fear of dementia, and of what is ahead with this terminal illness.

Blogging and other creative writing have helped me overcome my fear of criticism and critique, and encouraged me to be more open and honest, to look deeper within myself and sort all that 'inner stuff' out, including the emotional baggage. It's almost been like a clearing house, and has allowed me to see myself with an openness that was not easy to find before. Part of this, I suspect, is the fact that some people make comments that are complimentary, some are downright offensive, and others help you see there are other ways to view or feel about things. It is particularly cathartic too, writing it down for all to see.

Blogging and other writing have helped me build up a memory bank of my thoughts, life experiences and interactions with others, and have been and continue to be a vibrant channel of communication.

Blogging is a way of sharing and caring, for example there are many people caring for someone with dementia who follow this blog who tell me they find it very helpful in understanding how the person they are supporting feels. There are also people with dementia following this blog who say they find it helpful. I feel privileged and honoured they have shared some of their own lives with me. Sharing with others also helps me overcome my fears of the onslaught of the symptoms of dementia.

If you are worried about blogging being too technical, think of it as a diary or journaling, but one with a public audience. The reality is, it is simply words you write down about how you feel or what you are doing.

A dear younger friend of mine was admitted to a residential aged care home at the age of 55, with a number of serious health conditions including vascular dementia. My father-in-law was in the same nursing home, and very few days went by without us visiting them both, which continued with my friend after Dad died. I was also one of his legal guardians, and so had more than a friendship role in his welfare. In the first few weeks, even if we had been in earlier on that same day, this young friend would say he had not seen anyone for weeks, not because he hadn't, but because he had forgotten.

We implemented a diary, and whoever visited wrote a few notes about what had been talked about, or if they had taken him out for a coffee or to the movies, but it was something we had to do as he had lost the ability to write easily. When we were not there, apparently he took to reading this book to remind himself of what he'd been up and who had been to visit. It was like a living blog, but in hard copy, and helped him and his visitors keep informed about his life. So if you are scared to write a blog, even a private one that the public cannot access, then get an exercise book and start dictating or writing. It is not only a communication tool; it is very helpful for emotional healing.

Note: if you are afraid of what a blog is or if you could do it, in reality is just a website, so if you have done anything online, then you have the ability and easy access.

Fear is worth overcoming, and to have found blogging such a useful tool that helps me overcome the fear of dementia, and also offers me so many other positives, is truly wonderful.

The death of fear is simply finding the courage to do what you fear! I used to be afraid of writing and blogging! I used to be afraid of dementia, and now I am not.

Blogging and writing to capture memories

Blogging helps me to capture memories, and has become my personal history file, by way of words and stories embodying feelings and emotions. Blogging to capture my memories and thoughts has now become a significant tool in managing this disease, and one of the loves of my daily life. Speaking out through blogging, as a person with dementia, might also be the only way others will ever see positive changes in policy and funding, and so my new path as an advocate and activist for people with dementia, and through blogging, is to encourage others to use blogs to share their life stories. Mostly, with my words, I strive to break down the barriers and stigma around dementia.

My blog has become the journal of my life, my thoughts and my activities, ensuring my memories are retained, not only for my children later on, but for me right now. Other social media like Facebook and Twitter has become important too, as they offer other social connections and ways to record my world. All of them also have photographs, of people and events and activities, offering me yet another way to recall my world. On the days I can't remember a face when speaking on the phone, I go straight to one of these sites, as most people are now there with full frontals! We have indeed become a mildly narcissistic lot it seems!

My abilities are permanently damaged and my photographic memory is dead and buried! I read then I forget…I read then I forget…I read, I take notes, and then I forget…*I blog, and it is always there.* Computers and blogging have become my best friends as they constantly command my attention, edit for me, and perhaps more importantly push my brain to work hard every time I connect with them.

Dementia can represent the end of dreaming, a long and unforgiving one-way odyssey into obscurity, clouded in a thick and unforgiving fog. For me, *blogging has brought back the dreaming*. It inspires me to write more, creating a repertoire of my memories and personal history files, ensuring I leave some sort of record or legacy for my children to recall who I was and what I thought about. The excitement I felt with my first subscriber…and every time I get a new one, or some other feedback about something they have read…that I have written…something that also had meaning for them, or helped change their world in some small way, encourages me to keep going. It empowers me to rise above dementia and stay inspired and alive and I am certain it helps with neuroplasticity and creates new pathways for my brain to continue functioning.

Saul Alinsky wrote:

> We learn, when we respect the dignity of the people, that they cannot be denied the elementary right to participate fully in the solutions to their own problems. Self-respect arises only out of people who play an active role in solving their own crises and who are not helpless, passive, puppet-like recipients of private or public services. To give people help, while denying them a significant part in the action, contributes nothing to the development of the individual. In the deepest sense it is not giving but taking – taking their dignity. Denial of the opportunity for participation is the denial of human dignity and democracy.

A colleague and young friend Sam B sent me this quote, with the following comment:

> I thought it was really powerful and thought if you had not come across it already it might be something you could use in your writings about the importance of empowering people with dementia and ensuring their inclusion in all levels of

discussion about issues and service, support etc. that affect them.

People with dementia are still being left out of many of the conversations and events about them, and although this is changing, it is only changing slowly and, for my liking, far too slowly. It seems the many people without dementia who have been used to telling others, and us, what it is like for us, what is best for us, and how we cannot be included, often because we don't have the same capacity as others, are simply loath to give up their positions of power.

It is of course, much to do with why I speak out about living with dementia, to bring to light the stigma, discrimination, isolation and other negative experiences of living with dementia, as well as attempting to break down some of the other myths, including the biggest one that we can't live beyond dementia.

Megan Washington, a young iconic singer from Victoria, was interviewed about her TEDx talk on a programme I watched last year, where she revealed she has quite a pronounced stutter. Paul Grabowsky, a fabulous jazz musician, said when he interviewed about her talking about her personal and terrifying challenge of stuttering:

> It takes courage… And I wondered at the time if she realised how she might be helping a whole bunch of people…and to see someone, anyone really, who's got a challenge get up and talk about it publicly, and take that challenge head on, that's got to be a great example to people.

This resonated with me, and is part of the reason I write so candidly about my own experiences, not just of dementia, but in life. I have always loved reading autobiographies, and so, I suppose, blogging about one's own life is really just an autobiography in progress. And if it helps someone,

even just one person, then how much of a bonus is that…
Megan's TEDx talk has apparently helped hundreds of
people who stutter. How cool is that!

The scariest moment is always just before you start.

(Stephen King)

The optimist will always find a way to start; the pessimist will
always find a way to put it off. I am inherently an optimist,
I see the good in situations and people, and usually quickly
find a positive solution to everything that comes my way,
good and bad. One of my sayings is to ask myself (when
there is a problem), *has anyone died?* If they haven't, then
surely it (whatever 'it' is) is not really a problem.

The story of me being that kid in the room full of horse
shit is probably true, but I have also learned optimism and
practised it. Being an optimist has in part also kept me
blogging and writing. My blog post 'Reading and writing'[1]
has brought quite a variety of comments, and they are a
significant part of our lives. Comments inspire me to keep
writing, but also have kept me very grounded. So far, no
responses have yet put me off blogging most days, although
every negative one could be the start button for that (or stop
button?!). It included the following paragraph:

> Since blogging, and publishing a poetry book, I now feel
> like I am a writer, with readers. What a privilege to have
> people who enjoy my words and stories. The notion that
> I might give just one other person the simple pleasure I
> have always felt as a reader is awesome, a thrill so totally
> unexpected, mostly because I had never thought about
> it from the writer's perspective. To offer something up for
> another person to read, something I have not forced them to
> read is very fulfilling, even though it is as scary as hell. To

1   http://kateswaffer.com/2012/03/18/reading-and-writing

think I occasionally inspire someone to think beyond their own world, that I write something that someone else reads, that makes someone laugh (or a cry), is exquisitely inspiring to me as a writer, and a great honour.

Two blog followers commented via email to some blogs saying:

> Dear Kate, What a laugh! Firstly, that you think you're getting fat and, secondly, the funnies in your honest blog. I relate so well to today's words – and I'm still chuckling. The one about thermals was a scream, too. You DID draw a cartoon – with words! Keep up the good work and stay warm. Love MW.

Another email response said:

> Kate, you are not a real writer, and you should get over yourself, there's not a Shakespeare or Wordsworth anywhere in there yet. You are after all, just a blogger!! GB.

They did not send their comments to my blog, but both know me well enough to have my personal email address; I have chosen to copy them in here word for word (without their permission, but also without their names for privacy), as their comments well highlight the swings and roundabouts one must face when writing something that others can read. Some people love what we write. Some people hate it. Some people don't even care. As long as we love ourselves, I think we'll be okay.

There is a great book called *What You Think of Me is None of My Business* (Cole-Whittaker 1988), and I have tried to live by that mantra for a long time.

The reading of my blogs is a choice, and my blogs are not likely to ever be on the curriculum anywhere, but that is not why I write. And I do write, copious amounts of words each day, many of which will never make it here or anywhere else, but that is not the point.

I believe the blogs of people with dementia reinforce how important it is that many of us around the world living with a diagnosis of dementia have been speaking up about what is 'right for us' and what is hoped to be 'right for other people with dementia' whilst we are still able to have a say. Having our family help create a one or two pager for the nursing home staff to advise them of our likes, dislikes and preferred activities does not seem that helpful to me, and in many cases, by the time someone gets to aged care, this is what is done for us as most assume we are unable to communicate our own wishes, unable to give this information themselves. Blogging changes that, allowing us to ensure our wishes are written down, long before we lose capacity.

For me, writing is fun, it has become therapy, and it is the hard disc of my memory. Writing makes me a writer. Reading makes me a reader. Studying makes me a student. Working made me an employee (amongst other things). Cooking makes me a cook, but this almost always also makes people love me! My father always used to say, *the way to a man's heart is though his stomach*! I'm not so sure that is true, but it worked for Mum.

So I'll continue to be an optimist and will keep blogging and writing, until I have no words left inside my heart. I love your responses, no matter how or where you send them; the contrast of opinions is exciting and the more negative ones make me think more honestly, and the devil's advocates out there make me ponder and question more too. Of course I love the praise too; who wouldn't? Blogging and optimism are carefully bound together by food, readers and writers, all of us joining hands through our own experiences of life and love.

I've often considered stopping my daily blogging, and, in fact, did not blog as much as usual when completing this book, but the problem for me with that is it will remove the daily discipline of having to use my brain – the neuroplasticity workout, and I suspect reading a whole week or month's worth of my rambling musings will be too onerous for many of you. The other significant reason for daily writing is the therapeutic value it offers me. It is one of my non-pharmacological interventions for dementia, and one of my positive psychosocial interventions for dementia.

Like a daily Irbesartan tablet for someone with high blood pressure, or a jab of insulin for a diabetic, I suspect it is no longer optional. Ironically, the latest writing tools is an iPad, and is often referred to as a tablet!

Blogging is definitely an autobiography in progress, and it is also an intervention for dementia.

Advocacy as an Intervention for Dementia

Be yourself; everyone else is taken.

(OSCAR WILDE)

In an updated list of non-pharmacological and positive psychosocial interventions I use in an effort to delay the progression of the symptoms of dementia, I added advocacy to the lists. These lists, which I discussed in Chapter 28, evolve as I try new things, or as new symptoms appear and more specific interventions are needed. In many ways it is no different to modifying equipment for someone whose physical disAbilities are changing through disease or physical deterioration. Hence, I decided to write about advocacy, and why I think it is an intervention for dementia.

Advocacy is about owning your life, or helping someone else reclaim theirs.

As a non-pharmacological and positive psychosocial intervention, advocacy as an intervention for dementia works on many levels. As a self-advocate, it forces me to work my *little grey cells* harder, working on developing my neuroplasticity, helping to create new pathways in my brain.

To speak out about dementia means I have to read about and research it, research my own diagnosis, take notes, write speeches, practise speeches, and present in public. Speaking in public makes me work on speaking as well as I possibly can, pushes me to find ways to speak well and coherently, to maintain my dignity, one of the reasons I use a speech pathologist. It pushes me into new groups, providing 'colleagues', new contacts and new friends, adding to socialisation and significantly reducing isolation.

In line with Professor Martin Seligman's PERMA Principles (2011), it improves wellbeing by providing Positive emotions, Engagement, Relationships, Meaning and Achievement, thereby providing positive psychosocial value. It helps me to define myself by things other than the symptoms of dementia. I am therefore more than a person with forgetfulness, or odd behaviour, or a wanderer, or someone who is unemployed and therefore often undervalued. Advocacy gives me a reason to get up in the morning and work on my large list of interventions, in particular because it is meaningful.

Advocating for myself and others with dementia gives me a great sense of fulfilment when I feel like I have helped to bring about any change. This would be missing if all I did was focus on having dementia. Breaking down the stigma and ignorance in our community, within service providers and the nursing and medical communities also gives meaning to my life, as well as helping those of us living with dementia. Advocacy requires a significant amount of physical and emotional effort, and intent, and lots of new learning. It also can become our 'work', replacing the sense of loss from lost paid employment. These things have to be good for us!

In the disAbility sector, it is generally agreed people with disAbilities benefit greatly from learning how to advocate for themselves. The people with dementia whom I have met from around the world who advocate for themselves and for others all seem to have a sense of ease about their diagnosis, not that they are happy about it, but that they are actively trying to do something positive, and positively contributing to the dementia community. It unites us all, as well as gives us a global voice, making our individual efforts more powerful.

Beth Britton from D4Dementia today posted a blog titled 'Advocacy and dementia – A vital partnership'.[1] Obviously 'great minds think alike' with us both blogging on the same topic on the same day! My grandfather would have quipped back, saying 'and fools never differ!' It is definitely worth a read, but written from the perspective of people with dementia needing to have advocates speak for them, when they can't. This certainly reinforces how important it is that I have been speaking up about what is 'right for me' while I still can. I worked hard as an advocate for my father-in-law, and my friend Michael, thankfully with good results for both of them, but it is one very rough ride some days.

There are various definitions and aims of advocacy, and those listed below really resonate with me; I have clarified my own advocacy more fully as I continue to advocate.

On The Rights of Older People[2] site, the Institute for Family Advocacy and Leadership Development in Australia has defined advocacy as:

---

1   http://d4dementia.blogspot.com.au/2013/06/advocacy-and-dementia-vital-partnership.html
2   www.agedrights.asn.au/rights/whatis.html

the process of standing alongside an individual who is disadvantaged and speaking out on their behalf in a way that represents the best interests of that person.

Advocacy involves representing and working with a person or group of people who may need support and encouragement to exercise their rights, in order to ensure that their rights are upheld. It may involve speaking, acting or writing on behalf of another person or group, and differs from mediation or negotiation because these processes aim to reach a mutually acceptable outcome between parties. It also has no prescribed or clearly determined method. What constitutes advocacy will differ in different circumstances and according to the skills and needs of the individual or group, and may involve working against established or entrenched values, structures and customs, and therefore needs to be independent of service providers and authorities.

Advocates are not impartial because they work entirely from the perspective and interests of the other person or the self. Their role is to assist by representing the other person or person's wishes.

The common aims of advocacy are to:

- increase the person's control over goods and services
- overcome barriers that restrict opportunities
- ensure appropriate societal and service delivery responses
- protect human rights
- ensure a better quality of life
- be responsive to and emphasise individual needs and wishes
- be oriented towards outcomes for older people

- aim for empowerment of disadvantaged individuals and groups

- challenge stereotypes and stigma.

In 1994 Queensland Advocacy Inc.[3] defined advocacy like this:

> There are many definitions of advocacy and much debate exists regarding which one is the most appropriate to use. Having a definition of advocacy is necessary so that we have something to refer to, to check against and to encourage discussion about what we are doing. Action for Advocacy Development uses the following definition, which is based on the work of Dr Wolf Wolfensberger. Advocacy groups in Australia discussed this definition during a National Advocacy Workshop in Sydney in June 1994. Most of these elements were agreed on:
>
> Advocacy is speaking acting, writing with minimal conflict of interest on behalf of the sincerely perceived interests of a disadvantaged person or group to promote, protect and defend their welfare and justice by
>
> - being on their side and no-one else's
>
> - being primarily concerned with their fundamental needs
>
> - remaining loyal and accountable to them in a way which is emphatic and vigorous and which is, or is likely to be, costly to the advocate or advocacy group.

They describe five types of advocacy; Individual Advocacy, Citizen Advocacy, Systems Advocacy, Parent Advocacy and Self Advocacy. The Free Online Dictionary simply says:

---

3 http://qla.org.au/PDFforms/Advocacy%20Info.pdf

ad·vo·ca·cy (a-d v -k -s)

n. The act of pleading or arguing in favour of something, such as a cause, idea, or policy; active support.

Many days I talk about giving up my advocacy work, as I feel like it is not making a difference, or change seems too difficult to achieve. At these times, my dear husband nags me to keep going, or someone or something reinspires me to keep going. Many times it is a comment after a presentation, or a comment on my blog; most inspire and reinvigorate me. I may have seemed a little harsh about the voices of people with dementia missing from a conference a couple of years ago, but without them, a conference claiming to be giving a voice to people with dementia is simply increasing our social isolation and inequality if we are not on the plenary programme. It caused a groundswell of unrest leading to a tsunami of change that I believe will become cemented in history for people with dementia all over Australia; there will be no turning back and we will have a voice.

So, on the last day of this conference I was asked to speak about the new dementia advisory group being set up by Alzheimer's Australia, for people with dementia, run by people with dementia, with the support of Alzheimer's Australia. In the lift coming back to our hotel room, we met one of the new members of the research group I am on, and she complimented me on my presentation, and then, with tears in her eyes, told me it was the best presentation of the three days, and inspired her to keep going, to continue to advocate in memory of her partner who died from younger onset dementia. I felt deeply moved and humbled by this acknowledgement, but do know how she feels as so many have inspired me in the same way.

And so it seems, advocacy does work!

Below is my speech from this conference.

Thank you Rhonda Parker (CEO of Alzheimer's Australia WA) for inviting me to speak. I feel honoured and humbled to be representing all people diagnosed with dementia, of all ages, in Australia.

My thanks to Alzheimer's Australia Tasmania for hosting this conference, and for all your dedication and commitment to the event, and also for engaging the extraordinary Robyn Moore as MC, her love and passion for the lives of PWD and their families continues to inspire us all.

It is my great pleasure to be able to report further progress towards setting an Alzheimer's Australia Dementia Advisory Group, which Eric referred to this morning.

I have been advocating for this since meeting the Scottish dementia working group members in London at the ADI 2012 conference, and would like to thank Glenn Rees, the CEO of Alzheimer's Australia, and his wonderful team for working so hard to support this goal. I would also like to acknowledge Christine Bryden, the first person in Australia with dementia to speak up for us along with Peter Ashley and Richard Taylor.

So what are we going to achieve by having an advisory group for people with dementia, run by people with dementia? Firstly, there should be nothing about us without us. We also hope to ensure the human cost of dementia is more fully understood. Thank you to Eric and Joseph who shared with us their very personal stories this morning.

The group hopes to empower people with dementia, and to give them a voice about what it is that is important to them, and whether the current services available to them fit their needs. We want the group to be supported by all ages of people with dementia, from every pocket of Australia, and to represent every culture.

We hope to influence governments, service providers and the general community through raising awareness that we are still fully human, and with support, in the same way as any other person with a disAbility, and can live fulfilling lives contributing with purpose in meaningful purposeful ways.

We are thrilled to be setting this up now, perfect timing to be able to work with AAWA and ADI towards the 2015 conference in Perth, and it now gives me pleasure to invite Dr Glenda Parkin from Western Australia to say a few words. Glenda has a PhD in education, an honours degree in geology, and was a Principal at two prestigious colleges in Perth until retiring due to a diagnosis of younger onset dementia aged 57 in 2010. Glenda is going to welcome you to her beautiful state.

It is my very simple belief that people with dementia need to stand up and become advocates for each other and themselves, to argue in favour of our cause, for better dementia care, and for what is best for people with dementia. If we don't, others will keep deciding what we feel, and what is best for us.

CHAPTER 31

Volunteering as an Intervention for Dementia

Volunteering one's time, energy and talent to organisations can be a valuable service to not only those we volunteer for, but for ourselves. Studies have shown the financial and time costs associated with volunteering and the personal, organisational, client and community benefits generated by the volunteer activity are significant. However, overall, the main beneficiary of the volunteering is the volunteer. I've been volunteering most of my life, and have always found this to be true.

As an intervention for dementia, volunteering can be seen as a positive way to continue to thrive in our own community. When we can no longer do paid work, we can still contribute positively, redefining ourselves and providing an enhanced sense of purpose by doing things for others. Advocacy is also a form of volunteering, and many of the Alzheimer's organisations around the world are encouraging people with dementia to get involved.

As an intervention for dementia volunteering has a number of positive outcomes for people with dementia, and reduces many of the negative ones. My list below is not prescriptive nor is it exhaustive, and I'm sure you'll find more of your own:

- positive replacement for paid employment
- helps us to feel and stay physically and mentally engaged
- less of an emotional or physical burden on others
- still feel valued
- increases self-worth
- increases social inclusion and engagement
- reduces stigma
- reduces social isolation
- helping us maintain our skill sets
- can help us keep fit, depending on the volunteering activity
- encourages new friendships
- improves cognitive function
- improves the quality of life
- less support required from service providers
- may delay institutionalisation
- reduces care partner stress
- reduces psychological illness, e.g. depression, therefore
- increases wellness, and
- perceived longevity.

Working as a volunteer, for groups of people who are more marginalised than even people with dementia, helps me to keep my life in proper perspective. On the days I decide a pity party or PLOM (Poor Little Old Me) disease is all I can be bothered with, I usually find myself thinking about my homeless friends, some of whom live under a bridge. And there I am, sitting in the comfort of a beautiful home, with an amazing husband and kids... It is then that the pity party seems to be rather wasted!

CHAPTER 32

Dementia-friendly/ Accessible Communities

Dementia has a profound impact on the social welfare of the person with dementia, and the dementia-friendly communities initiatives have the potential to transform the quality of life of hundreds of thousands of people with dementia, supporting their independence and reducing pressure on the medical and social systems. Endorsed by the World Health Organisation, Belgium commenced with the Healthy Cities program, and was officially accredited in March 2011 as member of the Network of European National Healthy Cities Networks in Phase V. This has been successfully implemented in 25 cities in Belgium, and the Belgium Alzheimer's Association has helped to draft the Dementia-friendly Charter. Japan has done a lot of work in this space as well.

The determination by governments and Alzheimer's societies and organisations around the world to promote dementia-friendly communities and dementia champions still mostly supports the 'about them, without them' position, which has the potential to further stigmatise people with dementia. To date, only a few people with dementia have been included in the discussions, planning and decisions about what makes a community or organisation dementia friendly.

Australia has followed others, and, with many other countries, including the UK, is focused on becoming dementia-friendly. It is, of course, a noble pursuit.

A dementia-friendly community is a place where people living with dementia are supported to live a high quality of life with meaning, purpose and value. A dementia-friendly community must include people with dementia at every step, so it is important to set up a small Dementia Advisory Group of people with dementia, in every community or organisation planning to become dementia-friendly, to inform and guide a local or national Dementia Alliance which organisations and health care professionals can get involved in. The environment, including signage, noise levels, and location, must be dementia enabling, support for disAbilities must be provided for people with dementia in the same way as any other person with a disAbility, and the language you use must be respectful.

But first let's talk about what the term 'dementia-friendly' means, and by defining a few words relevant to this global movement or campaign.

To begin, being dementia-friendly means more than being friendly. From the perspective of people living with a diagnosis of dementia, it is less about being friendly, and so much more than awareness of what dementia is and how we are treated and supported. It is so much more than professionals and interested others (without dementia) working together to make *our* community more friendly and accessible.

It is more about:

• Respect

• Human rights

- Non-discrimination
- Full inclusion
- Our right to citizenship
- Autonomy
- Equality
- Equity
- Access
- Dementia Enabling Environments
- Support for disAbilities

Defining a few of these words puts the Dementia Friends movements into perspective, making them less about fundraising and organisations, and more about what the movement could be doing.

- *Friendly:* Characteristic of or behaving as a friend: *a friendly greeting; is friendly with his neighbors.* Outgoing and pleasant in social relations: *a friendly clerk.* Favorably disposed; not antagonistic.

- *Respect:* To feel or show deferential regard for; esteem or admire: *All the other scholars respect her.* To avoid interfering with or intruding upon: *Please respect my privacy.* To avoid violating: *I respected the speed limit throughout the trip.*

- *Equality:* The state or quality of being equal.

- *Accessible:* Easily approached or entered. Easily obtained: e.g. *accessible money.* Easy to talk to or get along with: *an accessible bank teller.* Easy to understand or appreciate: *an accessible library.*

- *Autonomy:* The condition or quality of being autonomous; independence.

- *Inclusion:* The act of including or the state of being included.

Supporting disAbilities and being dementia-friendly

Asking a person with dementia who is speaking at a conference to shorten their speech at short notice, simply to accommodate the insertion of an unexpected speaker ahead of them, is not dementia-friendly. Telling an audience that 10 per cent of the delegates are people with dementia, and then asking the audience to look around the room to see if they can pick them out is respectful and dementia-friendly. Making people with dementia stand up to be viewed like specimens, simply to make the same point, is offensive and not dementia friendly. Insultingly, this happened at an international conference in 2015, and I am sure if I had, in my keynote speech, asked the people with, for example, AIDS, cancer or schizophrenia to stand up to be applauded, most would have simply walked out!

Being dementia-friendly also means providing us with a more ethical post-diagnostic pathway of support, one that is enabling *and includes rehabilitation,* not disabling and which leads us only to aged care and death.

It means supporting us to remain employed, if that is our choice.

It also means using respectful language; that is, language that we, not people without dementia, find respectful, and if even a small group of us find terms such as 'sufferer' offensive, then no-one has the right to use them publicly. To do so means that you are not being dementia-friendly, or respectful.

It also means embracing the 10 Principles of Dignity in Care,[1] first developed in Birmingham in the UK and now part of a Dignity in Care Australia movement:

1   Zero tolerance of all forms of abuse

2   Support people with the same respect you would want for yourself or a member of your family

3   Treat each person as an individual by offering a personalised service

4   Enable people to maintain the maximum possible level of independence, choice and control

5   Listen and support people to express their needs and wants

6   Respect people's privacy

7   Ensure people feel able to complain without fear of retribution

8   Engage with family members and care partners as care partners

9   Assist people to maintain confidence and a positive self-esteem

10 Act to alleviate people's loneliness and isolation.

The myth that everyone with dementia has memory loss is wrong, and is being exacerbated by the use of the word 'memory' in so many activities. We have Memory Hugs, Memory Walks, Remember Me, and so on. I feel that the fact that all advocacy organisations begin with Alzheimer's, implying we all have Alzheimer's disease, is also unhelpful. I'd like to see Memory Hubs renamed Brain Health Hubs.

---

1   www.sahealth.sa.gov.au/wps/wcm/connect/public+content/sa+health+ internet/clinical+resources/clinical+programs/dignity+in+care

I'd like to see Memory Walks, which I have been told started as walks to remember those who had died from dementia, renamed as something less likely to keep the myth alive, perhaps something like Brain Health Walks. These terms would also work well with the Brain Health initiatives the advocacy organisations are now promoting.

The associations and organisations advocating for people with dementia and their care partners are sitting around tables, inviting guest speakers to present at events and teach others how to make their organisations and communities' dementia-friendly, and seemingly taking the notion of communities being dementia-friendly seriously.

In the work being done towards dementia-friendly communities, there are two pieces of the puzzle missing; one is the internal audit that needs to be done, inside their own organisations to see if they themselves are operating under the terms and guidelines of being dementia-friendly, and second is the full inclusion of people with dementia. I do not know of any truly dementia-friendly advocacy organisations. They generally are not fully inclusive of people with dementia, rarely have them on their Boards, and the consumer committees that have been set up to provide a consumer voice are predominantly made up of care partners, not people with dementia.

Thankfully this is changing, as the Scottish, European and Australian Dementia Working Groups made up entirely of people with dementia have set the trend. The Irish and Japan Dementia Groups have also been launched, modelled on what Scotland did in 2002. The Scottish group was ground-breaking, and set the example of what could and should be done.

Beyond these groups, not having *people with dementia*, not one person with dementia, at the table, at every single meeting about them, about what their needs are, being part of the conversations, is not dementia-friendly.

There is no way any country or community would be holding meetings or running events on what a gay or disAbled or Indigenous friendly community is without large numbers of those groups not only present, but leading the action.

Of course people with dementia rely on the support and services these organisations can provide, but not to their own detriment. Often we are 'used' in a patronising and tokenistic way, in order for them to say they have included us. We are used to help with fundraising, reported as 'sufferers' and 'victims' in order to elicit sympathy and support through fundraising for research. Research still mostly goes into finding a cure; even though some researchers openly and publicly admit they are further away from a cure than they were 10 years ago!

Furthermore, the literature does not read as dementia-friendly; it is still mostly about people with dementia, without them, and the language used is still inaccurate and offensive, and not in line with the current international guidelines. Dementia is not a mental illness (Ticehurst 2001), and as stated by Mukadam and Livingston (2012) in their article 'We're still the same people: developing a mass media campaign to raise awareness and challenge the stigma', it is a pathological or neurological illness. Second, the language being used remains stigmatising, negative and disempowering (Devlin, MacAskill and Stead 2007). These points are worthy of further consideration, as if the research literature, aiming to support decreasing stigma, is not accurate, and yet gets through the peer review process, using inappropriate, stigmatising and disempowering language, there seems little hope for progress or change.

The objective of a dementia-friendly community is to engage people with dementia in everyday life, and it is obviously meritorious. But, like cancer, dementia is not a single entity and it can be expected to affect any of a person's functions such as memory, language or understanding of space. A diagnosis of dementia exacerbates issues such as social inequality, stigma, isolation, loss of identity and discrimination. It also has the potential to set the person with dementia up to become a victim or 'sufferer', and their family caregivers to become martyrs.

It has significant negative emotional, financial and social cost and impact on the person with dementia, their families, and society. It disempowers, devalues, demeans and lowers self-esteem and very negatively impacts wellbeing and quality of life. Engaging people with dementia in the dementia-friendly projects must also mean employing them, and providing dementia-friendly communities, means people with dementia would become empowered to live their pre-diagnosis lives for as long as possible, and supported and enabled, allowing them to ignore the Prescribed Disengagement® given to them at diagnosis.

I have been uncertain that 'dementia-friendly communities' is the right phrase as I am worried it encourages division rather than includes people. Therefore, it is very important for the Alzheimer's societies and associations to ensure the dementia-friendly community projects work for people with dementia, and are not simply encouraging a tokenistic inclusion of people with dementia. They are working hard on dementia-friendly communities, some including audits on whether a community or organisation is dementia-friendly done by people with dementia. However, in supporting the dementia-friendly mantra, every Alzheimer's Society or Association must themselves be dementia-friendly, audited by people with dementia, and not by themselves or care partners. These audits, and the authentic voice of people with dementia deciding what is and what isn't dementia-friendly, are the missing pieces of the dementia-friendly community puzzle, and I believe, without them, no-one can claim to be dementia-friendly.

There are a range of issues important to understand and the critical part missing in research about dementia, and the organisations supporting people with dementia, is their authentic voice. Stigma is endemic in the literature, and the stigma and discrimination that still exists within the organisations advocating for people with dementia is increased by the language being used about them. It is clear from my lived experience, and reading of the literature, that stigma is still prevalent in the community, and amongst researchers, health care professionals and the associations advocating for and supporting us. The use of dehumanising language and the miniscule proportions of people with dementia in the research cohorts exacerbates stigma, and potentially means no community can be dementia-friendly. Contributing significantly to the stigma is the very low number of people with dementia in the conversations by the Alzheimer's organisations about them, on important topics such as the dementia-friendly projects.

If people with dementia only get 'used' for fundraising, or marketing or media opportunities, little will change. This type of 'inclusion' is tokenistic and patronising. The worth of any sector or agency (e.g. universities, Alzheimer's Societies or service providers) purporting to support this marginalised and stigmatised group, and the value of the research or projects being done about them without them, is flawed without the full inclusion and the authentic voice of people with dementia. It is important to remember that dementia is a social issue and not just a medical one.

There is much work to be done to assist the general public to understand and not be afraid of people with dementia, and to stop researchers and service providers from stigmatising us. In short, social action is needed to ensure we engage the wider community in understanding dementia and in that way reduce the social isolation, discrimination and stigma that people with dementia experience. We want to access services and to participate in the community the way everyone has a right to expect, and to have our disAbilities respected with acceptance, support and enablement.

Change is in the air and as the voices of people with dementia become stronger and louder, and more unified, through the work of a few organisations, including Dementia Alliance International, now the peak body for and voice of people with dementia, we will spread our wings and use our voices to ensure our basic human rights and disAbility rights are being met. Dementia-friendly must include us, and the organisations supporting us must weed their own back-yards through internal audits (not self-audits, but audits approved by people with dementia) before they start advocating and preaching to others what dementia-friendly means!

The one lesson I have learned, in the various positions I've held at Alzheimer's Australia – as a consumer advocate, Chair of the Dementia Advisory Committee and as consultant for six months ending in February 2015 – is that people with dementia function better if they are in smaller groups, in a dementia-enabling environment, and with disAbility supports. Therefore, it is important for advocacy organisations to set up Local Dementia Advisory

Committees or groups, to appropriately support people with dementia to have a voice in advocating for the needs and priorities of people with dementia in relation to service provision, information, support, education and dementia-friendly communities.

Any organisation or business can set up a Local Dementia Advisory Committee based on the example of the Dementia Working Groups around the world where members provide advice on policy and advocacy work, local programmes, and work to promote dialogue between those with dementia and service providers with a view to promoting a better understanding of their social and care needs.

Each Local Dementia Advisory Committee should aim to give a voice to people living with a diagnosis of dementia in that particular community, and to work specifically with their national, local or regional Alzheimer's office and the Local Dementia Alliance Committee on the dementia-friendly community initiatives. Of course, each community may be different based on local needs.

The Kiama Southern Dementia Advisory Group was the first of its kind in Australia and perhaps the world, and that group hopes other communities working towards becoming dementia-friendly will follow their model. Inclusion, at every step of the way, of people with dementia is imperative, and no community can become dementia-friendly without people with dementia at the heart of every conversation about them. I think it is important for communities working towards becoming dementia-friendly to role-model this group, which, although it is the first in Australia, was modelled on the Scottish Dementia Working Group, and the Australian Dementia Advisory Committee.

Expecting people with disAbilities caused by the symptoms of dementia to join a larger working group or

Local Dementia Action Alliance is, in itself, not dementia-friendly.

Whilst in national Dementia Working Groups or committees, membership works best if it is exclusive to people with dementia, in a smaller community, this may not be possible; for the Kiama Southern Dementia Working Committee, membership is drawn from Kiama and the surrounding local communities and includes people with dementia and care partners, but the 'brief' to the care partners or friends supporting the members with dementia is to allow them to speak for themselves or communicate in their own way and in their own time, not to speak for them unless they absolutely have to.

The following are some comments made after face-to-face meetings of the Alzheimer's Australia Dementia Advisory Group:

> I too thought the inaugural meeting was really worthwhile and it was so good to talk to other people in our situation (both those with dementia and those who stand by us) and how we will now hopefully take hopefully take a real part in the decision making that affects us.
>
> (Person with dementia)

> It will, I am sure, play a significant role now in mobilising our voice as people with dementia!
>
> (Person with dementia)

> I thought this new group would be a waste of time and money, but am thrilled to see that people with dementia are still so capable of speaking up, and how productive it has been.
>
> (Care partner, after Day 1 of our very first meeting)

The following is the most exciting feedback I have heard about the dementia advisory groups I've been involved in over the last two years:

> Until this meeting, I feel I have not spoken for myself for over 5 years!
>
> (Person with dementia)

> I found yesterday's meeting to be empowering, we both came away feeling that there are other people out there in a similar situation, and there is scope to contribute positively to the community.
>
> (Person with dementia, who attended with his care partner)

Based on the initiatives I have been involved with in Australia, and on what I have seen around the world, these are some of the key steps to becoming dementia-friendly/ accessible:

1 Establish a Local Dementia Advisory Group or Committee of people with dementia.

2 Establish a Local Dementia Alliance that will work together to make that community dementia-friendly, and that is guided by the Local Dementia Advisory Group.

3 Support local organisations and businesses to become dementia-friendly through making small changes that will have large impacts on the lives of people with dementia.

4 Encourage organisations and councils to have environmental audits.[2]

---

2   Such as DEEP at www.enablingenvironments.com.au.

5 Raise awareness of dementia through education and awareness campaigns.

6 Work with organisations to promote volunteering, employment and other meaningful engagement opportunities for people with dementia, and

7 Always, be mindful of the mantra, *nothing about us, without us.*

Dr Shibley Rahman shares a similar viewpoint as me on the notion that the term dementia-friendly might be more divisive than friendly and how best people with dementia can be part of these initiatives. In a very recent blog, 'Thought diversity is necessary for people living well with dementia to get a fair hearing',[3] he said this:

> I feel the insights from people living with dementia are essential in formulating the policy of how a community might be improved to improve the wellbeing, say perhaps in housing design. Such decisions are likely to be of a much higher standard in quality, in keeping with previous research, for example, from the Intelligence Advanced Research Projects Activity ('IARPA').
>
> This is not simply about hoping for the best, in getting a range of opinions, hoping that some opinions will gain legs. It is known that the first person to speak in a meeting often influences all subsequent opinions. The same effect could occur, for example, if a CEO of a regulator or a dementia charity talks at the top of a billing of a special event or world conference, with people living with dementia stuffed later down the programme (or even last).
>
> Or if there is a room of ten people, and one with a disparate view, the nature of joint decision making will mean

3 http://shibleyrahman.com/dementia-2/thought-diversity-is-necessary-for-people-living-well-with-dementia-to-get-a-fair-hearing

that the nine will tend to make the tenth person conform to a group view. This phenomenon is well-known from the studies of decision making in legal juries.

Exactly the same issues crop up again in the development of 'dementia-friendly communities' policy. While there are huge problems with this policy, possibly inadvertently causing division rather than true integrity and inclusion, it is possible the best we have currently both domestically and internationally. Change is often much easier from within, as Maya Angelou amongst others famously said.

I agree with him on this, and unless the dementia-friendly initiatives around the world start including us at the very beginning, and offer appropriate supports for our varying disAbilities to advocate for ourselves, I feel it is unlikely dementia-friendly will be achieved.

This is not rocket science, and the organisations promoting the Dementia Friends messages and campaigns need to start within so that they are walking their own talk. There is no need to 'sign up' to anything, just start.

Take baby steps. They are not expensive, and in fact many cost no money at all, but they can make a huge difference to the lived experience of people with dementia.

All too often, these campaigns and initiatives are simply being used as the new gateway to an organisation's own fundraising campaigns.

Below are the key first steps for any individual, organisation or community to consider:

- Always show respect.

- Use Dementia Language Guidelines. The best available are Alzheimer's Australia's.[4]

---

4   https://kateswaffer.files.wordpress.com/2015/08/alzheimers-australia-full-language-guidelines-20141.pdf

- Ensure any media you work with always refer to the Dementia Language Guidelines.

- Set up Local Dementia Advisory/Working Groups, in every community working towards becoming dementia-friendly. The Kiama Southern Dementia Working Group[5] is the only local group like this that I know of in the world.

- Employ people with dementia in this work, and in these campaigns, in the same way you would employ an IT expert for your IT issues.

- Focus on what we can do in your campaigns, not our deficits.

- Provide support for our disAbilities, in the same way you already do and are expected to by law for people with other disAbilities, such as wheelchair ramps and hearing loops.

Being dementia-friendly means including us

By not including us, the stigma, discrimination, myths of dementia and isolation are continued, and often by the very organisations and service providers claiming to advocate for us. Not one or two of us, but a lot of us, and this is why:

- People without dementia cannot really know what it means to live with dementia; we are the experts of the lived experience.

- People with dementia can inform people without dementia what it actually means [to us] to be dementia-friendly.

---

5   http://dementiaillawarra.com/dementia-friendly-kiama/

- So that it is no longer 'about us, without us'. This has become a catchphrase, a tick box for organisations, in the same way person centred care is seen in care plans, but not in action.

The Dementia Friends campaigns being run by advocacy and other organisations need to educate, not just raise awareness. They need to be respectful and empowering to people with dementia, and, very importantly, they need to promote, and use, respectful and empowering language.

If they engage with the media, and ask people with dementia to engage with the media, they must insist that the language being used is aligned with the most recently updated dementia language guidelines, as without using them, the media, and the organisation, will never be dementia-friendly.

Dementia Friends campaigns must never focus on our deficits. If our deficits are what are focused on, then we will never *transform the way the nation thinks, acts and talks about and towards the condition.*

Any organisation, wanting to work on something new, would contract or employ experts. People with dementia are the experts of the lived experience, and would [and should] significantly and positively impact this work.

In reality, especially in the earlier stages, people with dementia are simply living with disAbilities, that can be supported in the early stages of the disease. Yes, it is a terminal illness, and yes, it may not be a fun experience all of the time, but it is possible to live much better, for much longer, than the expectations and current perceptions.

We still have a lot to contribute to society, and our own lives. There are many groups of people working on their own Dementia Friends campaign, excited about what they might be able to achieve, how they might be able to improve the lives of people with dementia and our families, and talking about ways to support us to live beyond dementia, and to live in our communities for longer.

Everyone must start including us in this work. It is personal, and not including us simply means we have less chance of ever achieving this goal. If it's *about us without us*, it is not even remotely dementia-friendly.

And awareness is not education or training. I heard one private care provider recently say they are now a dementia-friendly organisation, because they are providing all of their staff with a 30-minute dementia awareness session. My reply was, 'So your staff, who are caring for people with dementia, are not yet trained in dementia?' Therefore, what they are doing, and using to promote themselves as dementia-friendly, is in reality what they should be providing for their staff already, as part of providing a professional dementia service. It is disappointing indeed when a dementia care provider does not automatically provide training in dementia for their staff, and then thinks a 30-minute awareness session entitles them to brand themselves as dementia-friendly. The campaigns, I believe, have a long way to go.

What's missing in the Dementia Friends campaigns?

Some key things currently missing in the dementia-friendly communities work and campaigns are:

- Each country, each city, each community working on becoming dementia-friendly must set up their local/ regional/city/country Dementia Working/Advisory Group. This is because every single community is different, and because the work must be led by people with dementia, not as it is now, which is by people without dementia.

- To be dementia-friendly themselves, advocacy organisations must start employing or contracting people with dementia, or an organisation like Dementia Alliance International, to work on their Dementia Friends campaigns. People with dementia should be treated with the same respect that any other consultant is, and paid for their expertise.

- They must also be audited on whether they are operating within their [which should be our] dementia-friendly guidelines, and being audited by people with dementia is the first place to start.

Join the global Dementia Friends movement

We ask that everyone join the global Dementia Friends movement, start your own local, regional, city or country Dementia Friends campaign, and support people with dementia, but please, always fully include us in this work.

And, finally, it should not be a marketing tool for organisations to promote themselves, which is what person centred care very quickly became.

By not ensuring that people with dementia at the heart of this work, the stigma, discrimination, isolation and loss of our most basic human rights are simply continued. It is also time that people with dementia were employed in this work as the experts, in the same way people with disAbilities or Indigenous people are being employed in the things they know most about, and that are about them. Most people without dementia cannot really know what it means to live with dementia, and by fully including us we can inform you on what it means to us to be dementia-friendly. It will stop it being 'about us, without us', we can educate and raise awareness, and this will empower others with dementia to also speak up for themselves.

Finally, when talking about dementia-friendly communities, I'd like to say how distasteful and discriminating setting up supermarkets with lanes specifically for people with dementia is. Whoever had this idea needs to rethink it. Whoever is promoting it needs to rethink it. Would we have mental health lanes, cancer lanes, HIV/AIDS lanes, venereal disease lanes, diabetes lanes, or Aboriginal lanes? It is offensive to label others by their disease or condition. In my opinion, this is no different to apartheid, when black Americans could not go into the same places as white Americans.

CHAPTER 33

Human Rights in Dementia and Aged Care

Safety is what we want for those we love, and autonomy is what we want for ourselves.

(KEREN BROWN WILSON)

The general content of this chapter was first published in 2014 in the *Australian Journal of Dementia Care* and discusses a consumer's perspective of human rights in aged and dementia care. I wrote that as a consumer, and as a person living beyond a diagnosis of younger onset dementia, one of 24,800 in Australia, and at the time with a mere 12 residential care beds interstate in Australia appropriate for someone my age.

I wanted to further open the Pandora's box into this issue, to promote and foster more conversations between all parties, and to encourage a deeper understanding of the issues we face, by those who are not being restrained against their will, that is, people without dementia, except for criminals. I have heard of very few age-appropriate facilities for people with younger onset dementia anywhere in the world, and to place younger people with dementia or other disAbling illnesses such as multiple sclerosis into aged care is a not only a breach of human rights, it is against many of the accreditation standards, at least in Australia.

Although it is presumably an easy topic, in light of the fact I believe our human rights are not being fully met in the care of people with dementia, I felt I should define them here. As defined by the Australian Human Rights Commission (2013), human rights:

> recognise the inherent value of each person, regardless of background, where we live, what we look like, what we think or what we believe. They are based on principles of dignity, equality and mutual respect, which are shared across cultures, religions and philosophies. They are about being treated fairly, treating others fairly and having the ability to make genuine choices in our daily lives. Respect for human rights is the cornerstone of strong communities in which everyone can make a contribution and feel included.

First, and importantly, I do recognise no-one goes to work intending to treat their patients or clients poorly, and that a significant percentage of the aged care sector (community, respite and residential care) is trying to do, and for the most part does do, the right thing.

However, we do have to question why people are being involuntarily restrained with physical or pharmacological restraints.

This is being done without the same stringent sanctioning guidelines required in the mental health sector, from which the guidelines for restraint being used in the aged and dementia care sector come under, and even though dementia is not a mental illness.

Australians and most others all around the world take considerable pride in their constitutionally defined and guaranteed civil liberties, yet our government and a number of institutions often abridge or completely ignore those rights when it comes to certain classes of people. Included in this group of people whose rights have been frequently ignored are people with dementia and people living in residential aged care.

All Australians are meant to be protected by the Universal Declaration of Human Rights, a significant document that took many years to design and get countries to sign up to. We speak up about the lack of rights of cattle in overseas countries, prisoners, asylum seekers, refugees, people with mental illness or disAbilities and many others, and yet until recently we did not speak up about the human rights of the infirmed elderly and people living with dementia. This declaration does not seem to apply to the health and aged care system. When we look at this declaration, we fall short for people who are chronically sick, aged and or who are diagnosed with dementia.

As a society, we should not be allowed to simply place a keypad on the front door, or the door of a specialised memory unit without adhering to some very strict guidelines. Yet, without any thought of basic human rights, we are locking people away.

In the majority of aged care facilities, the residents are not able to go outside of their own free will, often even those residing in a low-care facility. As a consumer, this looks like a blatant abuse of human rights. My father-in-law asked every time we went to visit him: 'Why have I been locked in prison?' and even in residential low-care he used to stand at the front door trying to escape. It seems we are allowed to be our own masters until we enter residential aged care, regardless of capacity.

Beyond the concept of being restrained with a keypad at the front door, other forms of restraint which could be deemed to be against a person's basic human rights include:

- antipsychotic and psychotropic medications

- assault

- chemical restraint

- withholding a person's possessions

- withholding a person's finances

- confining a person to a particular space, for example:

  » locking them in a house or room

  » using a tray table to keep them in a chair

  » using a particular type of chair so they can't get up on their own

  » using a particular type of mattress so they are unable to get out of bed

- physical restraint.

They are all gross forms of restraint and are often done without first trying to address the needs of the person with dementia; many times they are being used as a 'default' response to challenging situations rather than a last resort. Often, they are also done without consent.

The previous Australian Federal Government's 2012 *Living Longer Living Better* aged care reform package may have seen an improvement in the rights of people living in residential aged care facilities, but we may not see the fullness of its positive impact if the newly elected government does not continue with them. The overuse of antipsychotic medication and physical restraints as ways to manage 'behaviour' in aged care has been highlighted numerous times by the media recently (Australian Broadcasting Commission (ABC), Cannane 2013; ABC, O'Neill 2013; Belardi 2013b; Swaffer 2012a) and has shown us some appalling examples of abuse of residents living in aged care facilities. Of course, there are many examples of excellent care, but they do not often get air time in the media, and from my experience, they are still the exception, not the norm. The fact that the state I live in has declared dementia is no longer a health priority is beyond disappointing, considering our ageing populations and the global rate of diagnoses.

Since being diagnosed with dementia and joining the global campaign by people with dementia and others to help make things like person-centred care a reality, and advocating for what are the most basic of human rights for people with dementia, it fascinates me that we still have so far to go in achieving this. I constantly wonder why people with dementia have to fight so hard to be treated as whole and individual human beings, when virtually all other groups in our 'civilised' western society are accorded humane treatment.

What I find so curious about this is people with dementia have always been 'cared' for by an industry sector whose whole focus is to care for people who are sick or infirm!

They are trained to 'care', and yet many are not providing care that respects our humanity. Excellent person-centred care is the exception, not the norm. Dementia and aged care is definitely not sexy, and it is easier and cheaper to care for task needs rather than to care for the whole person. It seems to me these days this sector is mostly trained to treat the symptoms of disease, rather than the whole person.

Those who view involuntary restraint of any kind in aged care facilities or the acute hospital setting unquestionably and simplistically as a 'best interests' regime should be asking whether involuntary restraint, in fact, amounts to less favourable treatment. In terms of a person's subjective experience, and the fundamental rights and freedoms so central to a person's human rights, it certainly is. This treatment of people with dementia often will have serious, debilitating and stigmatising side effects.

Something that should be understood about involuntary restraint is that it usually involves a strongly felt and expressed resistance to the treatment, as opposed to an inability to express or make a decision due to an impairment relating to communication or cognition.

The expression usually manifests itself in 'behaviour', and there will often be good reason for a person's resistance, quite apart from the restriction on their autonomy.

It is worth noting that the restraint is always involuntary on the part of the person being locked up or restrained.

Being restrained – that is, locked in a 'secure memory unit', given drugs to make us compliant, or using physical restraints such as being strapped to the chair or bed – is done with the justification it is in our best interest, and that of those around us, and helps aged care or hospitals comply with their duty of care (avoid insurance claims!). As I see it, restraint is used because it is the quickest, cheapest and easiest way of providing 'care' with limited staff and funding. There is simply not enough funding, not enough staff and sometimes not enough willingness to manage the symptoms of dementia in a more humane way.

In many cases, it is worse than being locked in prison. The person with dementia has not broken the law or done anything wrong; they simply have a degenerative cognitive illness.

Many times I have written about human rights in aged and dementia care. There are many who agree with me, and then others who think I am too harsh on an industry doing its best to care for people with dementia and the aged, who have staff with low wages and organisations with limited funding to provide appropriate services. I was thrilled that Alzheimer's Australia National President Ita Buttrose AM has spoken so publicly about the lack of human rights in aged and dementia care (Belardi 2013a) and the abuse of physical or pharmacological restraints, not only because it was affirmation of what I have been saying for some time, but because someone with a high public profile was willing to take the risk of the public attack, who policy makers and those in power are more likely to listen to.

Aged care providers promote their facilities as being 'home away from home' and yet they are anything but that. We now know forcing institutionalisation of orphaned children and asylum seekers leaves them open to abuse, and yet we are institutionalising our elderly without due consideration of the 'to be expected' consequences leading to abuse and a lack of human rights. So how do I feel about the prospect of going into a residential aged care facility? It is currently the only place available for me in Australia if I need residential care, unless I can find a bed in a 12-bed facility for younger people south of Sydney, far away from my family and friends! I've been accused of being ageist for saying I feel like residential aged care facilities are not appropriate for me. I've been 'told' by many they are great places to live in, home-like and will be needed to reduce the load on my caring partner when the time comes. Of course, these same people have not lived in one.

It is fair to say that a significant percentage of the aged care sector – community, respite and residential care – is trying to do the right thing, but ultimately, we have to question why people are being involuntarily restrained. This is being done without the same stringent sanctioning guidelines required in the mental health sector, despite the same guidelines for restraint being used in the aged and dementia care sector. It is now time for consumers to step up to the plate, to speak up and speak out, and work together with like-minded people to bring about reform. It is clear we need radical change in the culture of ageing so that when our grandparents or parents (and eventually us) need to receive community, respite or residential aged care, we will thrive rather than decline.

We have a broken system, not broken people. The people who I know well or have had contact with working in aged and dementia care are some of the most caring people in the world.

The system needs to be fixed so that compassionate care workers can actually provide authentic person-centred care, not just go to workshops and talk about it.

We don't need new people, we need to radically transform the aged care system, and convert residential facilities into places where people want to live, and where people truly love to work. As the norm, not the exception, as it is now. Many people are now pledging to anyone who will listen about dignity in dementia care and how to reform the system. I'm joining them, in my own way, and hope together we can create a tsunami-sized wave of positive change. With some of the researchers and health care professionals now listening to and joining consumers collaboratively, I feel very confident we can and will make change.

People with dementia are not criminals. They have not done anything wrong or broken the law. They are diagnosed with dementia: an incurable terminal neurological disease.

Finally, the HALT study (2013) clearly states that the use of antipsychotics to manage 'behaviours of concern' is not only not best practice for dementia care, dementia is the one contraindication for these drugs in most cases.

I am delighted to close this chapter by saying I really do sense a huge and positive change in the aged and dementia care industry, and the dementia sector in general, as there does appear to be genuine and realistic positive change not only being talked about and advocated for, but actually in progress. The sector is really listening to those of us who are consumers, and really are wanting to engage fully with us, and to create change in their own organisations that is positive, life changing and affirming for us, and sustainable. I really do applaud them.

CHAPTER 34

There is Big Money in Dementia

This is the other reaction to dementia! In the middle of 2014, and for the first time in my life as a dementia advocate and speaker, it was not a pleasure to present at a conference, and it took me some time to recover emotionally, and to be able to talk more about it publicly. The final session of Day 1 of this particular conference was a panel discussion about the sexuality of people with dementia. During the question time I spoke up about being offended and distressed that on a plenary session like this, such a sensitive and personal topic was being discussed so publicly by people without dementia, and then, without including a person with dementia.

However, when I gave feedback to someone within the organisation, sadly, this was not only not well received, it ended with a public personal attack on me. I was bullied and had a finger pointed at me, and was very threateningly told 'Don't you dare hijack my conference', and in front of many witnesses. I was also publicly asked to prove my diagnosis, an extremely ignorant and offensive request.

It seems to me that many in the aged care and dementia sector are not in fact really about person-centred care, but more about *purse-centred care*, and some of the people working at the top are not really that well-informed about dementia at all. If people at the top of the chain in aged and dementia care cannot take criticism, from the very cohort they claim to care for, then we have no hope of improving the care of this vulnerable group at the coal face.

So often aged care providers have significant assets and dividends for shareholders, with annual reports that look more like marketing and promotional tools to encourage care partners to place people with dementia into their care homes, with lots of glossy pictures of happy residents walking in lovely gardens. Too often, the care inside those homes is less than optimum, and definitely not person-centred. It is based around the medical model of care, within an institution. And we all know that society no longer places children in institutions because we know they are subject to abuse.

There is, after all, big money in dementia.

Many aged care providers look and sound successful, so why would they change such a 'successful' formula.

There are also many private businesses now selling an array of things, from communication and engagement tools, care charts and pill dispensers, to miracle cures...some of them finding us online and swooping in on us. People with dementia have been so disempowered, and so isolated, that initially it often seems harmless and we are thrilled to be making new friends, until one day, it becomes clear we are being used, either to sell products such a 'miracle cures' to, or to promote a communication tool or some other product, sometimes simply through association.

People in private businesses, promoting products or services for dementia, are using people with dementia for their own credibility. Researchers have been doing it too, and Boards and organisations of advocacy organisations have been too. The tokenistic one person with dementia, used in all the marketing material, to prove they are not only selling something very 'useful for us', or their research is more valid, and that they, their research or their product is so wonderful they have included us. One person representing 47.5 million people; I don't think so!

There are even scammers using search tools for people with dementia on social media sites, who then send friend requests. Many of us have been caught, thinking it was a friend of a friend, or someone we have forgotten, only to find out after accepting their friend request, they are selling some miracle cure... We are a vulnerable group and very easy to target; and on top of that, before the internet, many of us were very socially isolated and now have embraced social media to make up for those others who are no longer in our lives.

Martin Luther King Junior once said, 'Our lives begin to end the day we become silent about the things that matter.'

I agree. My life matters. The lives of everyone I know, and who you know, matter. The lives of people with dementia all around the world matter, and it is important to keep speaking up about the things that matter to us all. I think we, as a group, have been used and abused, and it is rife at the moment due to the ease by which the internet makes it, particularly with scammers who are trying to sell us things like miracle cures.

It is important to keep getting up every time we are knocked down, just as at the conference I referred to earlier, it was important for me to turn up on Day 2 and give my presentations. What I have to say matters, and what other people with dementia have to say matters, not just to each other but to the people working to provide services and care for us.

Most people I meet at the conferences only have a job, because of people like me who have dementia.

Too often it also feels like many of the presentations accepted at dementia conferences are career-launching pads for academics and people working in the sector, or product-launching pads, and much more about self-promotion. A large proportion of the speakers are employees or associates of the conference convenors, which also seems a conflict of interest, and is not the optimum way to have unbiased presentation to delegates.

Self-promotion is a necessary fact of life, especially for organisations in such a competitive market, vying for the dementia and aged care dollar, but surely this should be through the usual advertising and marketing campaigns, not in the guise of a conference...or under the guise of providing person-centred care, or through 'befriending' people online or otherwise with dementia.

People are not yet used to people with dementia speaking up for themselves, but it is inexcusable that often when we do, we are at serious risk of being attacked, and very often by organisations and people who claim to be leaders in the field of dementia care. And it is even more inexcusable, in my humble opinion, that people with vested commercial interests, some in the aged care sector included, are so keen to make money out of such a vulnerable group of people.

CHAPTER 35

Nothing About Us, Without Us...

Never doubt that a small group of thoughtful committed citizens can change the world – indeed it is the only thing that ever does.

(ATTD. TO MARGARET MEADE)

Who's been missing in the dementia conversations?

You may think this is an odd question, but the people very often still missing in the conversations about people with dementia are the people with dementia. Yes, there is the one, sometimes even two, who are included at conferences or forums, or within an Alzheimer's Association or Society, but generally speaking, the inclusion is patronising and tokenistic, further supporting stigma and discrimination. There was for many months no representation on the World Dementia Council, not even one person with dementia. Most Boards of organisations advocating for people with dementia have no-one with dementia on their Board. They don't fully or even at all adequately include us in the planning of services meant for us for. It is still far too often about us without us.

Nothing about us, without us

The term *nothing about us, without us* was, as far as I could find, originally used in the disAbility sector about 30 years ago, and then people with dementia started using it about 15 years ago. I believe the Dementia Advocacy and Support Network (DASNI) was the first group in the dementia sector to use it, followed by the Scottish Dementia Working Group. When I was diagnosed, I heard it a lot, but rarely saw it in action. In many cases, this is still the case and so often people with dementia are left off of the committees and councils or the conferences and forums, about dementia, the very thing that affects them. However, it is still very often being used by people without dementia to give credibility to organisations and communities, without actually including us. It has lost its meaning.

Dementia Working Groups

Dementia Alliance International (DAI)

Dementia Alliance International (DAI) is the first global group, of, by and for people with dementia, where membership is exclusively people with dementia. Although DASNI was the first organisation set up by people with dementia for people with dementia (PWD), their membership did not remain exclusive to PWD. DAI is advocating for the voice and needs of people with dementia, and providing a forum for them of their own. There have been many with the dream or vision to set up a group like this, which we felt was needed as membership of DASNI had become two-thirds family care partners and only one-third people with dementia. Many people with dementia felt we needed our own voice, and I have no idea who was the first to have the idea, but many since my diagnosis had sowed the seeds, and so a group of us simply decided to do it. I make no claims to being the power behind the group, and am definitely not the person with the 'original' idea, but do know I am thrilled I am part of a group that made it happen.

DAI was launched on 1 January 2014 to promote education and awareness about dementia, in order to eradicate stigma and discrimination, and to improve the quality of the lives of people with dementia. They have recently collaborated with Alzheimer's Disease International (ADI) and have become the peak global organisation for people with dementia. I am a co-founder, and currently one of the co-chairs and the editor.

Our vision is a world where a person with dementia continues to be fully valued.

Our mission is to build a global community of people with dementia that collaborates inclusively. We aim to do the following:

- Provide support and encouragement to people with dementia to live well with dementia.

- Model to other people with dementia and the wider community what living well and living with purpose with dementia looks like.

- Advocate for people with dementia, and build the capacity of people with dementia to advocate for themselves and others living with the disease.

- Reduce the stigma, isolation and discrimination of dementia, and enforce the human rights of people with dementia around the world.

Dementia Alliance International is a group comprised of people living with dementia from all over the world representing, supporting, and educating others, and an organisation that provides a unified voice of strength, advocacy and support in the goal to achieve individual autonomy. Our website has a translator option, which does a very reasonable job of translating in most languages.

DAI is dedicated to the support of people living with dementia by people with dementia.

We are real people, diagnosed and living with dementia who no longer are willing to accept the continued absence of people with dementia from the decision-making processes and conferences that impact our lives every day.

DAI is dedicated to giving a global voice to people with dementia, of, by and for people with dementia.

Now is the time when 'Nothing about us, without us' is to become a reality.

People with dementia have been left out and left behind and now wish to be equal partners with others in our own care and treatment. The lack of self-advocacy for people with dementia is unacceptable in a world where full inclusion is the norm in other sectors to both change and progress. It is important to nurture the human potential of people with dementia, and DAI intends to provide a forum for that voice.

It is important to empower people with dementia to stop seeing themselves as 'victims' or 'sufferers' of a 'horrible' disease, and instead to focus on their assets and abilities. As a global community, it is up to us to reach out to others with dementia and to speak up and advocate for our basic human rights. What we can't do alone, we can do together.

The aim is to bring the community composed of those with dementia together as one strong voice to urge the government, private sector, and medical professionals to listen to our concerns and take action to address this urgent global crisis. It is our firm belief that working together, we will identify concrete action for implementation with the international community, and in the process, ensure our human rights are fully met.

We run monthly online cafes called Café Le Brain at two different time zones (currently the USA and Australia), have weekly online Support Groups also in many time zones, and run monthly educational Webinars called A Meeting of the Minds with topics specific to dementia and with guest speakers when possible. During Dementia Awareness Month 2014 we ran weekly Master classes, all available on our YouTube channel.

A full list of our online events and support services can be found on our website[1] and if you are a person diagnosed with dementia, you can become a member.[2]

Everyone else can subscribe to our weekly blog, or sign up to receive our newsletter.

Dementia Alliance International is working globally in collaboration with Alzheimer's Disease International towards ensuring that people with dementia are recognised under the UN Convention of the Rights of People with Disabilities. We have a long way to go, but my putting this onto the global stage in Geneva in March 2015 has not only pushed it more fully into the conversations, it has encouraged action. Words are, as always, mostly useless, unless they are followed up with action!

Dementia Advocacy and Support Network (DASNI)

The Dementia Advocacy and Support Network (DASNI) was opened on the Yahoo website on 8 November 2000 by Lorraine Smith, for people with early-stage dementia and their care partners. She registered it as a non-profit

---

1   www.infodai.org/events
2   www.infodai.org/membership

organisation in Montana. Peter Ashley from the UK gave an inspiring presentation on living with, not dying from, dementia. This ground-breaking work, which from my perspective when diagnosed had achieved very little real change for people living with dementia, most certainly paved the way.

The Scottish Dementia Working Group

The Scottish Dementia Working Group (SDWG) is a national campaigning group, run by people with dementia. The Working Group campaigns to improve services for people with dementia and to improve attitudes towards people with dementia. They are an independent voice of people with dementia within Alzheimer Scotland, and are funded by Alzheimer Scotland[3] and the Scottish Government. Membership is open to people with dementia.

They celebrated their tenth anniversary at the ADI 2012 London conference, my husband's and my first time attending this international conference, and we had the privilege and pleasure of meeting many of the members, and celebrating with them. I found them to be particularly inspiring, and I am sharing a little of an article I found on them from 2008.

Highlighted in the article are some of the reasons why we must all keep treading this path of awareness in our quest for better service provision and understanding; stories and policies written or told by us (people with dementia), not about us. We (people with dementia) must strive to take a leaf out of their book, and be at the centre of things with politicians and professionals too. The Scottish group were the trail blazers for the advocacy of people with dementia,

---

3   www.alzscot.org

in a very different way to DASNI, with more members, and better support. Fed up with having no voice on issues that affect them, a group of campaigners with dementia are making themselves heard in the corridors of power. Mary O'Hara reported in 'Bridging the gap' on 6 February 2008:

> Six years ago, James McKillop asked organisers of a care partners' conference in Scotland if he could attend and give a talk. When his request was refused, he posed as a photographer, gained entry and had his say anyway. McKillop laughs at his audacity now, but it kickstarted a career as an unconventional campaigner and marked him out as a new kind of advocate for people with dementia.
>
> 'They wouldn't let me go [to the conference] because I had dementia,' he recalls. 'That got me going. When you get a diagnosis, you're in a vacuum. You're put out the door and left there. Doctors and nurses have their unions, care partners have their groups, but there wasn't a single [user] group for people with dementia. I thought: "This is all wrong."'
>
> One year after he was denied access, McKillop attended the care partners' conference as a guest and official speaker. In the intervening 12 months, he had recruited a raft of like-minded people with dementia and helped set up the campaigning group, the Scottish Dementia Working Group (SDWG). Alongside the 60 or so people with dementia who signed up, he has managed to secure a voice for people diagnosed with dementia in the corridors of Scottish power.
>
> Fuelled by a righteous anger, the group has written to 'anyone we could think of', McKillop says. When he found out that for early diagnosis of Alzheimer's, the UK 'was propping up the bottom' of European league tables, he set about telling medical professionals and politicians that it was 'unacceptable'.

Follow the link for the full article.[4] It is worth reading.

However much ground work had been done by DASNI and the SDWG, when I was diagnosed I did not feel people with dementia had a voice, or were being given one, not in Australia, nor globally. Considering that ground-breaking work by DASNI and the SDWG, I am surprised and even shocked it took another ten years for others to follow, and that in many ways, we are only just now very much further along the path of people with dementia having their voices not only heard, but ensuring significant change, rather than the tiny baby step changes I was seeing. The fact that a group as important as the World Dementia Council has no-one with dementia (at the time of writing this) as a member says it all.

Like others, I will continue to speak out and advocate for aged and dementia care. Personally, I believe it is people with their own stories who have the most impact on achieving change. It turns the whole area of dementia into reality, not just words on a document or report.

Other Dementia Working Groups

The European Dementia Working Group in the footsteps of the SDWG was formed in 2012, with the support of Alzheimer's Europe, with Australia closely behind in 2013. The Irish Dementia Working Group was also formed in 2013, and during Dementia Awareness Month 2014 the Japan Dementia Working Group was launched and held its inaugural meeting. The Ontario Dementia Working Group is now in existence, and I have heard that a national Dementia Working Group is being planned for Canada and a few other countries.

4   www.guardian.co.uk/society/2008/feb/06/longtermcare.socialcare

The World Dementia Council

In March 2012, the UK Prime Minister published his Challenge on Dementia, setting out a number of key commitments to deliver major improvements in dementia care and research by 2015. As a result of this commitment and work, in 2014 we saw the World Dementia Council set up, focused on dementia now and into the future.

At the time of writing this book, Dr Dennis Gillings is the World Dementia Envoy, appointed by the UK Prime Minister in February 2014. The creation of this role was agreed at the G8 dementia summit in December 2013. Dr Gillings is a consultant to the pharmaceutical industry and founder of Quintiles. The envoy's role involves working with the newly created World Dementia Council and international experts to stimulate innovation and co-ordinate international efforts to attract new sources of finance, exploring the possibility of developing a private and philanthropic fund. He will also work with governments and stakeholders to assume a global leadership role in addressing the economic, regulatory and social barriers to innovation in dementia prevention, treatment and care.

During a public lecture that I was invited to in Australia in 2014, he began by saying, 'Perhaps people with dementia need to take to the streets in the same way the gay community did 30 years ago.' He suggested we need this zeal to fight dementia. If he was more active on social media he would have already heard us; we may not be walking with placards in front of a Parliament house, but we are speaking up loudly online, and at events, in droves.

During the lecture, Dr Gillings reviewed the global and Australian statistics, and then went on to outline the Five Priorities of the World Dementia Council as outlined briefly below. My notes were not perfect, but this gives you an idea of the lecture content.

Priority 1: Research

The first is research, and he said 'effective treatments, must be available, ASAP' and we need 'a faster pathway from early research to faster prescriptions' effectively 'speeding drugs to market'. He even met with the TGA (Department of Health, Australia) to ask them to participate more by allowing more drugs to market, and make it a priority.

Priority 2: Finance

Dr Gillings stated that dementia gets one-fifth of investment compared to cancer; funds are needed to accelerate clinical trials; the scale of investment is the key to success; goals are to identify and test the most promising drugs; and finally, he said, 'if we find the political will to make investments in research now, we will succeed' and that 'dementia must have the same support as other diseases'. There was quite a lot of discussion around research and funding, and he also talked about governments providing tax incentives or R&D credits to increase research investment; 'Pharma must believe the products will be approved' to want to continue investing in research into dementia.

Priority 3: Open science

Open research and big data was discussed, and the need for a structure around an easy one-step access to all data globally, including failed research so others knew not to go down those pathways. There is not enough data sharing, nor transparency between the research communities. In the question time, Christine asked him how did he anticipate encouraging academics to share emerging research, when often to the researcher, it was more about a career pathway, or about their own 'discovery'? A good question, which he agreed was one of the big challenges in the research community, that he really had no answer to.

Priority 4: Risk reduction

Dr Gillings said this is perhaps the most controversial in the research community, and again over dinner said this was one of his biggest challenges as too many researchers were not that interested in it as the data does not support it (yet). However, he made the comment that risk reduction included improving health and lifestyle factors, and that 'common sense must prevail', and there was data to support this approach in other areas, so why not dementia. He also said it was the 'short-term hope – until *drugs* become available!'

Priority 5: Care

The fifth priority of the World Dementia Council is care for people with dementia, and it needs to include technology and new models of care. He talked about the value of robots, showing a short clip of some in use and of technology being used to remind people to take medication, to help them up after a fall, and even to shower them. He said, 'whilst technology and robots can assist in care, they do not replace face to face care', although I suspect robots are on their way to replace humans in the care of people with dementia and the elderly, as many countries already do not have the young workforce to provide it. I suspect there will be times when there is no alternative, and no care is not preferable to a robot providing some care.

Dr Gillings closed with a few things, including stating the target of a cure or disease-modifying drugs is the goal, by 2025. He also said, 'advocacy and awareness is the key to progress'. I definitely agree with that last comment.

Now is the right time for people with dementia to make contact with the universe, to remind people on earth we do exist…and that we are a form of intelligent life!

Perhaps, as Dr Gillings suggested, we will have to make some placards and rally in front of Parliament Houses all over the world to make people sit up and take notice.

CHAPTER 36

Love, Gifts, Dementia and Dying

In the book *Julie and Julia* by Julie Powell there are two beautiful lines that sparkle. Julie talks about a girlfriend and marriage, and how no-one would be 'good enough for her – not smart enough, not kind enough, with no gift to match her percolating laugh, her voice that can spread its champagne bubbles throughout a room of strangers' (2005, p.88). Then of her parents' separation and reuniting, she says, 'they stayed together anyway, not because they were the "marrying kind", but because they'd worked like hell and "loved each other more than they'd hurt each other"' (p.92). What wonderful insight, what beautiful words to say of a friend or parent. These are things for us all to think about and aspire to, and a peek into the souls of others, with wisdom beyond the mundane. Being the girl who spreads champagne bubbles through a room full of strangers…wow, who wouldn't want to be like that?! The notion of loving someone more than you are hurting them is so powerful.

Writing about this means I will have some hope of retaining some of the richness of my life and reading adventures, and some chance of the optimism required to keep going, to keep working against the symptoms of dementia. The effort of reading, and then writing about reading, whether by blogging or by attaching coloured Post-it Notes, covered with words, all over the book, is still meaningful and worthwhile, and keeps my glass half full when I forget to look at it this way. The message from these words is that love and laughter must always be at the top of my tree.

I realise how fragile everything in life is, and how comfort begets taking something or someone for granted. I took great comfort in my abilities, my memory, my intellect and my ability to be empathetic and sympathetic. My dear husband, with his unconditional support and belief in me, helps me get through the difficulties, and to accept the ever-evolving 'Kate'. In knowing every time I stumble, he will be there, every text, every call, every email, every question and every proclamation, I can go on. I find great joy in that and wrap my thoughts of his constant and undying faith and love for me around me.

Thinking about dying has a way of making me even more philosophical and to think a lot about life and in general. In 2012 my youngest son Charles said he thought I was the happiest he has ever seen me. This was and still is in spite of the obvious sadness and grief I have openly displayed about my illness. A few years ago, a lecturer from a university said he had never seen me look so 'well', not in the physical sense, but in a holistic sort of way.

Perhaps this is the real gift of illness and dying. I think being diagnosed with a terminal disease, and then spending time focused on what you want for what is left of your life, is significant. It allows you to put life in perspective. It stops you worrying about the small stuff, about whether it is too hot or raining today, about whether the coffee served up in the cafe is perfect or not. Who really cares about these things if you might not even be there tomorrow to enjoy a coffee or, for me, remember you have even had one!

Love, laughter and spending time with your loved ones is all that seems to matter and the opportunity of this gift of illness and dying gives the freedom to be true to yourself.

Perhaps that truth is the real gift, and the inner peace that comes with it. You, and I, will all live until we die.

A Final Word on Resilience and Memory

Children act in the Village as they have learned at home.

(SWEDISH PROVERB)

Those things that hurt…instruct.

(BENJAMIN FRANKLIN)

The past… You leave it all behind, but it always stays with you.

(RAELENE BOYLE)

Whatever you do, don't let anyone steal your joy… Not even Mr Dementia.

(KATE SWAFFER)

I thought I'd close with a few words about resilience and memory. Resilience refers to an individual's capacity to successfully adapt to change and stressful events in healthy and constructive ways. Building resilience is important if we are to strengthen our capacity and our skills in order to reduce emotional and mental health problems, and this is important for those of us with dementia, or those of you caring for someone with dementia. It is a skill worth developing as it will give you the ability to overcome obstacles of your past, it will help you recover from health, career or relationship setbacks and reach your full potential, and it will help you cope with a difficult 'present'.

We all need to encourage personal responsibility, accept more and question less. Accept yourself and your past. Accept your future, which if you have dementia, or someone you love has it, needs doing, or it will cripple you.

Become more mature. Forgive your parents. Forgive your ex-husband or wife. Make a choice to live your life with passion and reason, to make a difference in at least one other person's life, if possible every single day, and to live every day as if it really is your very last.

You might ask, is it really possible to make a choice to become more resilient? I believe it is. Life is no more than a series of experiences, some good and some bad. I honestly believe you can make a choice in how you react to them. If you are feeling down, you may make the choice of not going to work today, or of refusing an invitation out with friends or colleagues. However, if your best friend arrived on your door step from another country, your first time together for 20 years, you would pull yourself together, stop wallowing in your misery and enjoy the time together. I really believe that if you take a truly honest look in the mirror, you will eventually see this. If, initially, it is too hard to look within, start on your best friend, or quietly and anonymously analyse the actions of someone you do not get on with. It will be easier in the beginning, to be honest, weeding someone else's garden! Then when you get used to doing this, try it on yourself.

Next time you have the opportunity; have a look at a small child's response to falling off a bike and skinning their knee. If their mother is not there, and especially if their friends are present, they will not end up in tears or dolefully complain about the pain. Follow them and watch their response when their friends are gone and their mother is there. Yes, they will cry for her attention, to make sure she notices their pain. When my children were young they often complained of being too tired for homework or housework, or way too alert or busy to go to bed…but always found renewed energy and enthusiasm if I suggested a trip to the beach or the movies. Eventually they worked it out! They stopped me playing these games, but they did learn the lesson of making a choice. They learned to take personal responsibility, not just for their actions, but also for their reactions and emotional responses.

When faced with a new problem, my standard reaction is to ask myself 'Will it be a problem in a year?' If it will, then I work on a solution to fix it, rather than spending time bemoaning the problem. It if won't be a problem in a year, then I simply forget about it. I guarantee if you spend no time lamenting or worrying over it, you will barely be able to remember it that night, let alone the next day. So get rid of PLOM (poor little old me) disease. It will only cause you to spend more time with negative thoughts, less time with positive and constructive ones. Live, love and laugh more, worry less.

My father's advice to me many times during my childhood was to 'only act grown up when you absolutely have to'. I spent many years trying to take his advice, but was so wrapped up in myself and in being serious, I could not truly understand it. I suggest you behave more like a 'mature' child, with uncomplicated naivety and freshness. Let the simple things take your fancy, do good deeds, love more openly and spend more time thinking about things other than yourself. Our versions of events (our memories) are more often an expression of what we want to have been true, rather than what was true. They can become a way of justifying our behaviours, of not getting go of our past. So let go of your hang-ups, let go of the past injustices you believe others may have inflicted upon you and look for wisdom and lessons in every situation. Find ways to forgive and move on and in doing so help yourself and your loved ones to become resilient.

I've also been wondering, how does losing memories impact on a person with dementia, if they can't remember their loved ones, or the love felt and expressed by them? When I was nursing in a secure dementia unit, many family members used to say they felt desperately sad their loved one could not remember them, and often not recall their face or name, or even a glimpse of how they knew the person, and it always seemed much sadder for the family member than the person with dementia. Now that I'm wearing the shoes of the person with dementia, I'm not so sure…

Given my penchant for blogging, it should come as no surprise I think the greatest gift of the practice has been the daily habit of reading what I had written on that day some time earlier; not only is it a remarkable tool of introspection and self-awareness, and my memory bank, but it also illustrates that our memory *is never a precise duplicate of the original (but) a continuing act of creation* (Cartwright 2010) and how flawed our perception of time is; almost everything that occurred a year ago appears as having taken place either significantly further in the past or significantly more recently. Rather than a personal deficiency of those of us ensued by this tendency, however, it turns out to be a defining feature of how the human mind works, the science of which is at first unsettling, then strangely comforting, and altogether intensely fascinating.

That's precisely what acclaimed BBC broadcaster and psychology writer Claudia Hammond explores in *Time Warped: Unlocking the Mysteries of Time Perception* (2012), a fascinating venture into the idea that our experience of time is actively created by our own minds and how these sensations of what neuroscientists and psychologists call 'mind time' are created. As disorienting as the concept might be, it is also strangely empowering to think that the very phenomenon depicted as the unforgiving dictator of life is something we might be able to shape and benefit from. I also think it is interesting to think about when questioning if memory is important. Hammond writes:

> We construct the experience of time in our minds, so it follows that we are able to change the elements we find troubling – whether it's trying to stop the years racing past, or speeding up time when we're stuck in a queue, trying to live more in the present, or working out how long ago we last saw our old friends. Time can be a friend, but it can also be an enemy. The trick is to harness it, whether at home, at work, or even in social policy, and to work in line with our conception of time. Time perception matters because it is the experience of time that roots us in our mental reality. Time is not only at the heart of the way we organize life, but the way we experience it. (Hammond 2012, p.7)

But there is a lot to think about when it comes to memory, and perhaps, after all, it is not as important we all want to believe.

As Anne Basting's book title says, perhaps we should all just *forget memory!* (2009).

For being at the end, I thank you. Anyone who can make it thus far probably deserves a medal!

CHAPTER 38

Proof People with Dementia Can Live Beyond a Diagnosis of Dementia

Finally, to let you know it really is possible for some of us to live beyond a diagnosis of dementia, this is a list of my current professional activities:

- Honorary Associate Fellow in the Faculty of Science, Medicine and Heath, University of Wollongong, Australia, 2015 – current

- Consultant, Alzheimer's Australia, 2014–February 2015

- Educator, dementia and aged care, 2010–current

- Published author and poet

- International speaker on dementia

- Alzheimer's Disease International Board member

- Alzheimer's Disease International; Scientific Panel, conference 2015 committee

- Global Action on Personhood (GAP) in Dementia, core member, 2014 – current

- Cognitive Decline Partnership Centre, Steering Committee member, 2015 – current

- Supporting GPs and Practice Nurses in the Timely Diagnosis of Dementia project, Steering Committee member, 2014 – current

- National Dementia in Hospitals Program, Advisory committee member, 2014 – current

- Kiama Dementia Advisory Group, Honorary member, 2014 – current

- International Consortium for Health Outcomes Measurement (ICHOM), working group member for international dementia protocols

- Dementia Alliance International; Co-founder, Chair, Board member and Editor
  A global advocacy and support group, of by and for people with dementia, now also supported by Alzheimer's Disease International as the peak body for people with dementia.

- Alzheimer's Australia (National office), Consumer advocate

  » Chair, Dementia Advisory Committee (AADAC)

  » Past member, National Consumer Advisory Committee (NCAC)

  » Co-chair, Consumer Dementia Research Network (CDRN), plus various committees

- Alzheimer's Australia SA (AASA), Consumer advocate, Dementia Champion:

  » YOD reference group

> » AASA Consumers Alliance

> » Dementia-friendly Communities Working Group

- Dignity in Care Australia Action group, member, SA Health:

> » Education and conference 2015 subcommittee

> » Dementia Champion

- Consumer Representative with Health Consumers Alliance South Australia:

- Author and manager of consumer website and daily blog,[1] an online space committed to meaningful dialogue with a wide range of stakeholders about the critical issues impacting a person living with a diagnosis of dementia and their loved ones.

  Current readership at time of writing this book of 40,000+ per month; in 2012, my blog was also archived in the PANDORA Collection of the State (SA) Library and National Library of Australia.

  It is currently listed in the following educational institutions and organisations as a resource:

> » Edinburgh University, MSc Dementia: International Experience, Scotland

> » Murray Alzheimer Research and Education Program, Ontario, Canada

> » NSW Department of Health Dementia Care Resource and Training Network

> » Flinders University, Bachelor Applied Science (Physiotherapy): Rehabilitation of Degenerative Neurological Disorders

---

1 http://kateswaffer.com

» University of Tasmania, Wicking's Understanding Dementia Massive Open Online Course (MOOC) and Bachelor of Dementia

» YoungDementiaUK

- The Big Issue South Australia, fundraising committee and originator of their major annual fundraising event, The Big Lunch, held at the famous Adelaide Central Markets.

My professional credentials

2014 Masters of Science in Dementia Care, Distinction, University of Wollongong

2010 Bachelor of Psychology, University of South Australia

2009 Bachelor of Arts, Writing and Creative Communication, University of South Australia

2005 Certificate of Small Business Management, Business SA

1989 Graduate Diploma in Grief Counselling, University of Ballarat

1987 Chef diploma: Australian Cuisine, Regency Park TAFE

1977 Nurses training, Whyalla Hospital SA

Selected presentations

Since 2009, I have given more than 600 presentations at forums, conferences, dementia study days, aged care service provider training sessions and meetings, Federal Australian Government, Department of Health SA, consumer groups, AGMs, Church groups, and various other groups. I have listed a few of them below.

2015 United Nations World Health Organisation first Ministerial Conference on Dementia, Geneva, plenary speaker

Dignity in Dementia Care 2015, plenary speaker

Parliamentary Summit on Dementia, Canberra, plenary speaker

Alzheimer's Disease International, plenary speaker

National Dementia Congress, plenary speaker

2014 NZ Biennial Conference, keynote speaker

Australian Government Minister's Dementia Advisory Group forum, Melbourne, invited speaker

ADI Puerto Rico, presenter, and invited speaker (for opening ceremony)

Dignity in Dementia Care, Adelaide, invited keynote speaker

2013 ADI Taipei, presenter (April)

Australian Government, Minister's Dementia Advisory Group forum

Canberra Psychology Private Australia Inc, Tenth National Congress, guest speaker

2012 Adelaide Fringe Festival performance, *My Unseen Disappearing World* (four performances)

Caladenia Dementia Care, keynote speaker

Dementia Collaborative Research Centre Research Forum, invited guest speaker

Aged & Community Services SA & NT, *Demystifying Consumer Directed Care*, invited guest speaker

Alzheimer's ACT, Dementia Network Education 2012, invited guest speaker

2012 Alzheimer's Disease International, London, presenter and invited speaker

Thinkers in Residence, *The Science of Well-being* Conference, invited speaker

Future Faces of Dementia, NZ Biennial Alzheimers Conference, keynote speaker

2011 Alzheimer's Australia *Fight Dementia Campaign* Rally, invited speaker

WordCamp Gold Coast, invited keynote speaker

2009 Helping Hand RN and Carers training day, invited guest speaker – my very first dementia speaking event!

Publications and books

Swaffer, K. (2014/2015) 'Reinvesting in life after a diagnosis of dementia.' *Australian Journal of Dementia Care 3*, 6, 31–32.

Swaffer, K. (2014) 'Dementia and Prescribed Disengagement®.' *Dementia 14*, 1, 3–6.

Swaffer, K. (2014) 'Dementia: Stigma, language and dementia-friendly.' *Dementia 13*, 6, 709–716.

Swaffer, K. (2014) 'Human rights in residential aged care: A consumer's perspective.' *Australian Journal of Dementia Care 3*, 1, 9–10.

Swaffer, K. (2013/2014) 'Introducing the Australian Dementia Advisory Committee.' *Australian Journal of Dementia Care 2*, 6, 13–14.

Swaffer, K. (2013) 'Driving and dementia.' *Australian Journal of Dementia Care 2*, 4, 17–18.

Swaffer, K. (2011) 'My unseen disappearing world.' *The Big Issue 389*, 16–19.

Swaffer, K. (2008) 'Dementia: My new world.' *Link Disability Magazine 17*, 4, 12–13.

Swaffer, K. (2012) 'You Live Until You Die.' In P. Willis and K. Leeson (eds) *Learning Life from Illness Stories*. Mt Gravatt, Qld: Post Pressed, Chapter 7, pp.90–101.

Swaffer, K. (2012) *Love, Life, Loss: A Roller-coaster of Poetry*. Richmond, SA: Graphic Print Group.

Swaffer, K. (2010) 'Kate.' In *Words That Shine*. Magill: Poetry and Poetics Centre, University of SA, pp.11–16.

Swaffer, K. (2009) 'Slipping Away.' In C. Short *et al.* (eds) *Stratosphere*. Magill: Piping Shrike, University of SA, p.85.

Clark, S., Jones, H., Goldney, R., Swaffer, K. and Cooling, P. (1993) 'A support group for the bereaved.' *Crisis 14*, 4.

I was also a major contributor to a book by Dr Sheila Clark, *After Suicide: Help for the Bereaved*, 1995, published by Michelle Anderson Publishers, Australia.

Honours and awards

2015 Dementia Leader of the Year, Dementia Services Development Centre University of Stirling International Dementia Awards 2015, Winner

2015 Emerging Leader Disability Awareness, National Disability Awards 2015, Winner

2015 Australian of The Year Award 2016, South Australian Finalist

2015 Australian Association of Gerontology, Recognition of Achievements in 2014 at University of Wollongong

2015 Dignity in Care Achievement Award 2015, Outstanding Individual Contribution to Dignity in Care, Inaugural Winner

2015 Bethanie Education Medallion Award, Winner

2015 University of Wollongong, Community Engagement Award, Winner

2015 University of Wollongong, 2015 Alumni Award Social Impact Category, Runner up

2014 University of Wollongong, Master's of Science in Dementia Care, Distinction

2012 My blog 'Creating life with words: Love, Inspiration and Truth' was archived in the PANDORA Collection of the State (SA) and National Library of Australia

2012-13 Patron for The Visitors, a play about Younger Onset Dementia, Urban Myth Theatre Group and ECH Residential Aged Care, based on my personal story

2008 Bachelor of Psychology University Merit Award, University of South Australia

2008 Lifetime Golden Key Membership, University of South Australia

Dementia:
A Brief Summary

A CLOUD OF FOG

The end of dreaming
A long and remorseless
One way odyssey into obscurity
Clouded in a thick and
Unforgiving fog

(KATE SWAFFER 2012)

This book is less about what dementia is, and focused more on my experience of being diagnosed, and learning to live beyond it. Those of us living with dementia are in fact the experts, through the lived experience. However, this chapter with support from Alzheimer's Australia and the Mayo Clinic briefly describes dementia and the current (at the time of publishing) available pharmacological treatments for it.

Dementia is an umbrella term, in the same way fruit is for all types of fruit, with subcategories even within the main categories. It is a syndrome, rather than a single disease. In simple terms, dementia is the gradual deterioration of functioning, such as thinking, concentration, memory, and judgement, which affects a person's ability to perform normal daily activities. Brain function is affected enough to interfere with the person's normal social or working life. It is a terminal illness. There are approximately 130 types or causes of dementia; Alzheimer's disease is one type of dementia, and is the most common type making up between 60 and 80 per cent of all dementias.

Dementia occurs primarily in people who are over the age of 65, or in those with an injury or disease that affects brain function. While dementia is most commonly seen in the elderly, it is not a normal consequence of the ageing process. Dementia over the age of 65 is known as 'older onset dementia', and under the age of 65 as 'younger onset dementia'. All age groups go through the stage of early onset dementia. Alzheimer's and all other dementias are currently incurable. The available drugs can alleviate some of the symptoms but are generally only recommended for some of the dementias of the Alzheimer's type, but they don't cure the disease. There is currently no treatment for all other types of dementia.

Doctors diagnose dementia if two or more cognitive functions are significantly impaired. The cognitive functions affected can include memory, language skills, understanding information, spatial skills, judgement and attention. People with dementia may have difficulty solving problems and controlling their emotions. They may also experience personality changes. The exact symptoms experienced by a person with dementia depend on the areas of the brain that are damaged by the disease causing the dementia.

With many types of dementia, some of the nerve cells in the brain stop functioning, lose connections with other cells, and die. Dementia is usually progressive. This means that the disease gradually spreads through the brain and the person's symptoms get worse over time.

There are a few very rare forms of inherited dementia, where a specific gene mutation is known to cause the disease. In most cases of dementia, however, these genes are not involved, but people with a family history of dementia do have an increased risk.

Certain health and lifestyle factors also have been shown to play a role in a person's risk of dementia. People with untreated vascular risk factors including high blood pressure have an increased risk, as do those who are less physically and mentally active. Up-to-date and detailed information about dementia risk factors is available on the Your Brain Matters and other websites.[1]

The incidence of dementia worldwide is rapidly increasing and currently there are estimated to be 47.5 million people diagnosed with dementia in the world (WHO 2015). Alzheimer's Disease International[2] (ADI) reported 'there are 7.7 million new cases of dementia each year, implying that there is a new case of dementia somewhere in the world every three seconds'. Is it estimated more than 342,800 Australians are currently diagnosed with dementia effects (Alzheimer's Australia 2015), including one in four over the age of 85, making it the second leading cause of death in Australia,[3] and an estimated 1800 new diagnoses per week, and as the incidence of dementia rises globally, the rate and scale at which it is currently escalating has forced governments to make it a health priority; in Australia it was made the 9th Health Priority in 2013.[4]

The commissioning of the World Dementia Council in 2014 indicates the seriousness with which governments are taking dementia, but the initial exclusion of people with

1   www. yourbrainmatters.org.au
2   Alzheimer's Disease International 2013.
3   https://sa.fightdementia.org.au/about-dementia/statistics
4   www.aihw.gov.au/dementia

dementia from membership of this Council indicated the continuation of an 'About us without us' mindset, and they have since invited one person with dementia to join the Council, with a second person with dementia to be announced in 2016.

- There are over 130 types or causes of dementia; dementia is a syndrome.

- There is estimated to be a new diagnosis of dementia worldwide every three seconds.

- There are now 47.5 million people with dementia worldwide.

- There are currently 342,800 people with dementia in Australia.

- Dementia is a terminal progressive degenerative chronic illness.

- There is treatment for some of the dementias of the Alzheimer's type, no treatment for all of the others, and no cure.

- Alzheimer's disease is a dementia; it is one of over 130 types or causes of dementia.

- Dementia is not a normal part of ageing.

- Dementia affects all ages.

- People diagnosed with dementia still experience isolation, stigma and discrimination.

- People diagnosed with dementia feel a sense of shame and humiliation.

- The language used to refer to people with dementia in the media, the health care system and in research is disrespectful.

Largely attributed to the late Tom Kitwood is the phrase 'If you've met one person with dementia, you've met one person with dementia.'

Therefore, it is not possible or even appropriate to think one person can adequately represent the 47.5 million people with dementia around the world.

This book and my advocacy seek not to do that either, but to explore my personal experience of living with dementia and improve awareness, services and care.

Some of the most common forms of dementia

Alzheimer's disease

Alzheimer's disease is the most common form of dementia, accounting for around two-thirds of cases. It causes a gradual decline in cognitive abilities, often beginning with memory loss. Alzheimer's disease is characterised by two abnormalities in the brain – amyloid plaques and neurofibrillary tangles. The plaques are abnormal clumps of a protein called beta amyloid. The tangles are bundles of twisted filaments made up of a protein called tau. Plaques and tangles stop communication between nerve cells and cause them to die.

Vascular dementia

Vascular dementia is cognitive impairment caused by damage to the blood vessels in the brain. It can be caused by a single stroke, or by several mini-strokes occurring over time. These mini-strokes are also called transient ischaemic attacks (TIAs). Vascular dementia is diagnosed when there is evidence of blood vessel disease in the brain and impaired cognitive function that interferes with daily living. The symptoms of vascular dementia can begin suddenly after a stroke, or may begin gradually as blood vessel disease worsens. The symptoms vary depending on the location and size of brain damage. It may affect just one or a few specific cognitive functions. Vascular dementia may appear similar to Alzheimer's disease, and a mixture of Alzheimer's disease and vascular dementia is fairly common.

Lewy body disease

Lewy body disease is characterised by the presence of Lewy bodies in the brain. Lewy bodies are abnormal clumps of the protein alpha-synuclein that develop inside nerve cells. These abnormalities occur in specific areas of the brain, causing changes in movement, thinking and behaviour. People with Lewy body disease may experience large fluctuations in attention and thinking. They can go from almost normal performance to severe confusion within short periods. Visual hallucinations are also a common symptom.

Three overlapping disorders can be included with Lewy body disease:

- dementia with Lewy bodies
- Parkinson's disease
- Parkinson's disease dementia.

When movement symptoms appear first, Parkinson's disease is often diagnosed. As Parkinson's disease progresses, most people develop dementia. When cognitive symptoms appear first, this is diagnosed as dementia with Lewy bodies.

Lewy body disease sometimes co-occurs with Alzheimer's disease and/or vascular dementia.

Frontotemporal dementia

Frontotemporal dementia involves progressive damage to the frontal and/or temporal lobes of the brain. Symptoms often begin when people are in their fifties or sixties and sometimes earlier. There are two main presentations of frontotemporal dementia – frontal (involving behavioural symptoms and personality changes) and temporal (involving language impairments). However, the two often overlap.

Because the frontal lobes of the brain control judgement and social behaviour, people with frontotemporal dementia often have problems maintaining socially appropriate behaviour. They may be rude, neglect normal responsibilities, be compulsive or repetitive, be aggressive, show a lack of inhibition or act impulsively.

There are two main forms of the temporal or language variant of frontotemporal dementia. Semantic dementia involves a gradual loss of the meaning of words, problems finding words and remembering people's names, and difficulties understanding language. Progressive non-fluent aphasia is less common and affects the ability to speak fluently. Frontotemporal dementia is sometimes called frontotemporal lobar degeneration or Pick's disease.

Is it dementia?

There are a number of conditions that produce symptoms similar to dementia. These can often be treated. They include some vitamin and hormone deficiencies, depression, medication effects, infections and brain tumours. It is essential that a medical diagnosis is obtained at an early stage when symptoms first appear to ensure that a person who has a treatable condition is diagnosed and treated correctly. If the symptoms are caused by dementia, an early diagnosis will mean early access to support, information and medication should it be available.

What are the early signs of dementia?

The early signs of dementia can be very subtle and vague and may not be immediately obvious. Some common symptoms may include:

- progressive and frequent memory loss
- confusion
- personality change
- apathy and withdrawal
- loss of ability to perform everyday tasks.

What can be done to help?

At present there is no cure for most forms of dementia. However, some medications have been found to reduce some symptoms. Support is vital for people with dementia and the help of families, friends and care partners can make a positive difference to managing the condition.

Treatments and drugs

Most types of dementia can't be cured. However, doctors will help you manage your symptoms. Treatment of dementia symptoms may help slow or minimise the development of symptoms, and this information on the treatments and drugs current at the time of writing this book is from the Mayo Clinic.[5]

5   www.mayoclinic.org/diseases-conditions/dementia/basics/treatment/con-
20034399

- *Cholinesterase inhibitors.* These medications – including donepezil (Aricept), rivastigmine (Exelon) and galantamine (Razadyne) – work by boosting levels of a chemical messenger involved in memory and judgement. Side effects can include nausea, vomiting and diarrhoea. Although primarily used to treat Alzheimer's disease, these medications may also treat vascular dementia, Parkinson's disease dementia and Lewy body dementia.

- *Memantine.* Memantine (Namenda) works by regulating the activity of glutamate. Glutamate is another chemical messenger involved in brain functions, such as learning and memory. A common side effect of memantine is dizziness. Some research has shown that combining memantine with a cholinesterase inhibitor may have beneficial results.

- *Other medications.* Your doctor may prescribe other medications to treat other symptoms or conditions, such as a sleep disorder.

My thoughts on medication

Finally, a few points or issues for you to consider if you or someone you care for are being prescribed medication for the symptoms of dementia or 'behaviours of concern'. However, you should always seek the advice of a medical doctor. Do not consider what I have written here as medical advice.

- It is important to know that the latest guidelines for the use of antipsychotics for people with dementia is that dementia is the *one contraindication* for these drugs, unless there is a mental illness such as schizophrenia or severe psychosis.

- Agitation, anxiety, or other 'behaviours' are not a valid reason to be taking antipsychotic drugs; read more about the de-prescribing of antipsychotics in the HALT study.[6]

- All drugs can have side effects, some of which may make the person's symptoms worse.

- Always ask the doctor why the drug is being prescribed and what side effects might occur.

- A drug which is useful may not continue to be effective indefinitely because of the progressive changes to the brain caused by dementia.

- Do not expect immediate results. Benefits may take several weeks to appear particularly with antidepressants. Discuss this with the doctor.

- It is important that treatment is reviewed regularly. All new medications should be reviewed regularly, at a minimum of three monthly.

- If you are a legal guardian of someone who no longer has capacity, then the health care provider has a legal obligation to ask you before prescribing with any medication, especially antipsychotics.

- Keep a record of all medications, including alternative medications and vitamin supplements.

- Take this record to all medical appointments.

- Many people with dementia take a number of medications for different symptoms. It is important to

---

6   www.dementiaresearch.org.au/index.php?option=com_dcrc&view= dcrc&layout=project&Itemid=142&pid=249

discuss with the doctor any impact that medications may have on each other.

Reminder: always seek the advice of a medical doctor. If you are not happy with one doctor, do seek the advice of another.

A list of *resources* can also be found in Appendix 2.

Resources

Dementia Alliance International

If you are a person living with dementia, I recommend you join Dementia Alliance International (DAI): www.joinadi.org. I am a founding member, and in 2016 will continue to be the editor as well as co-chair.

DAI provides online weekly support groups and a monthly Café Le Brain in numerous time zones, as well as educational Webinars on topics of interest and many other services. We have a weekly blog and a monthly e-news update, with members in many countries, and a translation button on the website. Whilst anyone can subscribe to our blog or newsletter, membership is exclusive to people with dementia.

Our vision is simple: A world where a person with dementia continues to be fully valued and fully included.

To learn more about what dementia is or of other services for people with dementia and family care partners please go to your own country's Alzheimer's Association or Alzheimer's Society, and the services they can provide.

Dementia links

For Australians, Alzheimer's Australia offers support, information, education and counselling. Contact the National Dementia Helpline on 1800 100 500, or visit their full website at www.fightdementia.org.au.

Please visit your own country's Alzheimer's Association or Society for local information, services and support, although I have added a few of them in the list of links below.

This list, although not exhaustive, is of websites and resources many will find useful. You will find a more detailed explanation of dementia, and the numerous types of dementia, and resources in your own country.

Alzheimer's Disease International is the peak body for people with dementia and their family care partners. www.alz.co.uk

Dementia Alliance International is the peak body of people with dementia. www.joinadi.org

'Dementia: my story.' What it felt like not long after diagnosis. https://www.youtube.com/watch?v=9ZUyIRq5DAs

'What is that? (Τι είναι αυτό).' A *must*-watch short movie; there is no question it will change you. https://www.youtube.com/watch?v=mNK6h1dfy2o

'If we could see inside other's hearts: life in 4 mins.' A profound look at life in four minutes. https://www.youtube.com/watch?v=Wl2_knlv_xw

The late Dr Richard Taylor. An amazing man and personal friend who lived with dementia, and was a pioneer advocate for people with dementia. www.richardtaylorphd.com

I CAN! I WILL! An 'Ideas Library' for PWD, their families, professionals, associations and others. www.alz.co.uk/icaniwill

Alzheimer's Australia. www.fightdementia.org.au

Younger Onset Dementia Association. www.youngeronset.net

Alzheimer's New Zealand. www.alzheimers.org.nz

Alzheimer's Society (UK). www.alzheimers.org.uk

YoungDementia UK. www.youngdementiauk.org

Alzheimer Society of Canada (Canada). www.alzheimer.ca/en

Alzheimer Europe. www.alzheimer-europe.org

Fisher Center for Alzheimer's Research Foundation. www.alzinfo.org

Frontier: Neuroscience Research Australia. www.neura.edu.au/frontier

National Alzheimer's Association (USA). www.alz.org/index.asp

The Mayo Clinic Alzheimer's Blog. www.mayoclinic.org/diseases-conditions/alzheimers-disease/expert-blog/CON-20023871

Moving your soul: a different way to be with Alzheimer's. A wonderful tribute to loved ones by care partners. www.movingyoursoul.com

'I am one. The dignity song' by Amanda Waring. www.youtube.com/watch?v=VjLCQ0VTVQ0&feature=youtube_gdata_player

Dementia and Elderly Care News. Loads of excellent research articles on this site. www.dementianews.wordpress.com

Books of related interest

Basting, A. (2009) *Forget Memory.* Baltimore, MD: The John Hopkins University Press.

Doidge, N. (2012) *The Brain That Changes Itself.* Melbourne, Vic: Scribe Publications.

Doidge, N. (2015) *The Brain's Way of Healing.* London: Allen Lane

Ellison, P. and Sandlant, V. (eds) (2012) *The Good, The Bad, The Brilliant: Lessons from the Journey of Living with Dementia.* Adelaide, SA: Resthaven Incorporated.

Hughes, J.C., Louw, S.J. and Sabat, S.R. (eds) (2006) *Dementia: Mind, Meaning, and the Person.* Oxford: Oxford University Press.

Innes, A. (2009) *Dementia Studies: A Social Science Perspective.* London: Sage Publications.

Lipton, B. (2005) *The Biology of Belief: Unleashing the Power of Consciousness, Matter and Miracles.* London: Hay House Inc.

Rahman, S. (2014) *Living Well With Dementia: The Importance of the Person and the Environment for Wellbeing.* London and New York: Radcliffe Publishing.

Rahman, S. (2015) *Living Better with Dementia: Good Practice and Innovation for the Future.* London: Jessica Kingsley Publishers.

Sabat, S. (2001) *The Experience of Alzheimer's Disease: Life Through a Tangled Veil.* Oxford: Blackwell Publishers.

Seligman, M. (2011). *Flourish: A Visionary New Understanding of Happiness and Well-being.* New York, NY: Free Press.

Swaffer, K. (2012) *Love, Life, Loss: A Roller-coaster of Poetry.* Kelbane, Richmond, SA: Graphic Print Group.

Tanzi, R. and Chopra, D. (2012) *Super Brain: Unleashing the Explosive Power of Your Mind to Maximize Health, Happiness, and Spiritual Well-Being.* New York, NY: Harmony Books.

Taylor, R. (2007) *Alzheimer's from The Inside Out.* Towson, MD: Health Professions Press Inc.

Walker, R. (2012) *The Five Stages of Health.* London: Transworld Publishers.

Willis, P. and Leeson, K. (2012) *Learning Life from Illness Stories.* Mt Gravatt, Qld: Post Pressed.

References

ABS (2010) in Australian Institute of Health and Welfare (2012) *Dementia in Australia*. Cat. no. AGE 70. Canberra, ACT: AIHW.

Albom, M. (1997) *Tuesdays with Morrie*. New York, NY: Doubleday.

Algase, D., Moore, D., Vandeweerd, C, Gavin-Dreschnack, D. and IWC (2007) 'Mapping the maze of terms and definitions in dementia-related wandering.' *Aging and Mental Health 11*, 6, 686–698.

Alinsky, S.D. (1971) *Rules for Radicals: A Pragmatic Primer for Realistic Radicals*. New York, NY: Vintage.

Alzheimer's Australia (2012) *Exploring Dementia and Stigma Beliefs: A Pilot Study of Australian Adults Aged 40 to 65 Years*. Available at https://fightdementia.org.au/sites/default/files/20120712_US_28_Stigma_Report.pdf, accessed on 24 November 2015.

Alzheimer's Australia (2013) *What is Dementia?* Available at www.fightdementia.org.au/understanding-dementia/what-is-dementia.aspx, acessed on 11 October 2015.

Alzheimer's Disease International (2011) *World Alzheimer's Report 2011: The Benefits of Early Diagnosis and Intervention – Executive Summary*.

Alzheimer's Disease International (2013) *Dementia Statistics*. Available at www.alz.co.uk/research/statistics, accessed on 9 December 2014.

Alzheimer's Society of Ireland (2008) *Media Guidelines to Dementia Language: Dementia-friendly Language*. Available at www.alzheimer.ie/about-us/news-and-media/media-guidelines-to-dementia-language.aspx, accessed on 21 April 2014.

Anonymous (2009) *Poetry Aims to Help Cut Dementia Problem*. Darlington (UK): Newsquest (North East) Ltd.

Anstey, K., Wood, J., Lord, S. *et al.* (2005) 'Cognitive, sensory and physical factors enabling driving safety in older adults.' *Clinical Psychology Review 25*, 1, 45–65.

Australian Broadcasting Corporation (ABC), reporter Steve Cannane (2013) 'Nursing home residents are being sedated.' *Lateline*. Transcript: www.abc.net.au/lateline/content/2013/s3808604.htm.

Australian Broadcasting Corporation (ABC), reporter Margot O'Neill (2013) 'Assaults in nursing homes go unreported.' *Lateline.* Transcript: www.abc. net.au/lateline/content/2013/s3735328.htm.

Australian Government (1992) Disability Discrimination Act. Available online at www.comlaw.gov.au/Details/C2005C00204, accessed 16 September 2015.

Australian Human Rights Commission (2013) *What are Human Rights?* Available at www.humanrights.gov.au/about/what-are-human-rights, accessed on 1 December 2013.

Austroads (2012) *Assessing Fitness to Drive.* Available at www.austroads.com.au/ drivers-vehicles/assessing-fitness-to-drive.

Barca, M.L., Thorsen, K., Engedal, K., Haugen, P.K. and Johannessen, A. (2014) 'Nobody asked me how I felt: Experiences of adult children of persons with younger onset dementia.' *International Psychogeriatrics 26*, 12, 1–10.

Bartlett, R. (2014) 'The emergent modes of dementia activism.' *Ageing and Society 34*, 623–644.

Basting, A. (2009) *Forget Memory.* Baltimore, MD: The John Hopkins University Press.

Batsch, N., Mittelman, M. and Alzheimer's Disease International (2012) *World Alzheimer's Report 2012: Overcoming the Stigma of Dementia.* London: Alzheimer's Disease International.

Belardi, L. (2013a) 'Buttrose decries aged care standards.' *Australian Ageing Agenda.* Available at www.australianageingagenda.com.au/2013/05/01/ buttrose-decries-aged-care-standards, accessed on 11 October 2015.

Belardi, L. (2013b) 'Call to entrench human rights in aged care.' *Australian Ageing Agenda.* Available at www.australianageingagenda.com.au/2013/06/14/ article/Call-to-entrench-human-rights-in-aged-care/APIAVMJXVT.html, accessed on 11 October 2015.

Benbow, S. and Jolley, D. (2012) 'Dementia: Stigma and its effects.' *Neurodegenerative Disease Management 2*, 2, 165–172.

Bier, N., Macoir, J., Gagnon, L., Van, d. L., Louveaux, S. and Desrosiers, J. (2009) 'Known, lost, and recovered: Efficacy of formal-semantic therapy and spaced retrieval method in a case of semantic dementia.' *Aphasiology 23*, 2, 210–235.

Bredesen, D. (2014) 'Reversal of cognitive decline: A novel therapeutic program.' *Aging 6*, 9, 707.

Bright, P., Moss, H.E., Stamatakis, E.A. and Tyler, L.K. (2008) 'Longitudinal studies of semantic dementia: The relationship between structural and functional changes over time.' *Neuropsychology 46*, 8, 2177–2188.

Bryden, C. (2006) *Dancing with Dementia: My Story of Living Positively with Dementia.* London: Jessica Kingsley Publishers.

Burack-Weiss, A. and Ebrary (2006) *The Caregiver's Tale: Loss and Renewal in Memoirs of Family Life.* New York, NY: Columbia University Press.

Burgener, S. and Berger, B. (2008) 'Measuring perceived stigma in persons with progressive neurological disease: Alzheimer's dementia and Parkinson's disease.' *Dementia 7*, 1, 31–53.

Burns, K., Jayasinha, R., Tsang, R., Brodaty, H. (2012) *Behaviour Management – A Guide to Good Practice*. Dementia Collaborative Research Centre, University of South Wales. Available online at www.dementiaresearch.org.au/images/dcrc/output-files/328-2012_dbmas_bpsd_guidelines_guide.pdf, accessed on 15 September 2015.

Carel, H. (2008) *Illness: The Cry of the Flesh*. Stocksfield, UK: Acumen.

Cartwright, R.D. (2010) *The 24 Hour Mind*. Oxford: Oxford University Press.

Civil Aviation Safety Authority (2013) *Pilot's Exams and Licenses*. Available at www.casa.gov.au/scripts/nc.dll?WCMS:STANDARD::pc=PC_90004, accessed on 11 October 2015.

Clark, S. (2013) 'Review: Learning life from illness stories'. *Australian Family Physician 42*, 4, 252.

Clasper, K. (2014) 'Time to raise awareness of dementia again.' Blog post, *Living well with Lewy Body Dementia*, 20 April. Available at http://ken-kenc2.blogspot.com.au/2014/04/time-to-raise-awareness-of-dementia.html, accessed on 21 April 2014.

Cole-Whittaker, T. (1988) *What You Think of Me is None of My Business*. New York, NY: Jove Publishing.

Collins, C. (2009) 'A Dying Mind: the profound losses of early onset dementia.' *Link Disability Magazine 18*, 3, 22–24.

Croot, K. (2009) 'Progressive language impairments: Definitions, diagnoses, and prognoses.' *Aphasiology 23*, 2, 302–326.

Dean, E. (2011a) 'Stigma and dementia care.' *Nursing Older People 23*, 5, 12.

Dean, E. (2011b) 'Workloads and staff levels hamper dementia care.' *Nursing Older People 23*, 5, 6.

Dementia Awareness Month (2014) 'Media Release: Diagnosis of younger onset dementia has life changing impact on families.' Available at http://sydney.edu.au/medicine/cdpc/documents/media-releases/media-release-yod-workshop-3-Sept-14.pdf, accessed on 13 October 2015.

Devlin, E., MacAskill, S. and Stead, M. (2007) '"We're still the same people": Developing a mass media campaign to raise awareness and challenge the stigma of dementia.' *International Journal of Nonprofit and Voluntary Sector Marketing 12*, 1, 47–58.

Dictionary.com (undated) 'Myth.' Available online at http://dictionary.reference.com/browse/myth, accessed on 15 September 2015.

Doidge, N. (2012) *The Brain That Changes Itself*. Melbourne, Vic: Scribe Publications.

Doidge, N. (2015). *The Brain's Way of Healing: Stories of Remarkable Recoveries and Discoveries*. London: Allen Lane.

Elias, N. (2001) *The Loneliness of the Dying*. New York, NY: Continuum Publishing.

Etymonline.com, Online Etymology Dictionary (undated) 'Myth.' Available online at http://www.etymonline.com/index.php?term=myth, accessed on 15 September 2015.

Fossum, K. (2003) *Don't Look Back.* London: Vintage Imprints.

Frankl, V. (2006) *Man's Search for Meaning.* Boston, MA: Beacon Press.

Frittelli, C., Borghetti, D., Iudice, G. *et al.* (2009) 'Effects of Alzheimer's disease and mild cognitive impairment on driving ability: A controlled clinical study by simulated driving test.' *International Journal of Geriatric Psychiatry 24,* 232–238.

Garand, L., Lingler, J., Conner, K., and Dew, M. (2009) 'Diagnostic labels, stigma, and participation in research related to dementia and mild cognitive impairment.' *Research in Gerontological Nursing 2,* 2, 112–121.

Gaukroger, M. (2014) 'Update: The emotion involved in caring for a parent with Younger Onset Dementia.' *Dementia News.* Available at http://dementiaresearchfoundation.org.au/blog/update-emotion-involved-caring-parent-younger-onset-dementia, accessed on 13 October 2015.

Goffman, E. (1963) *Stigma: Notes on the Management of Spoiled Identity.* Englewood Cliffs, NJ: Prentice Hall.

Hagens, C., Beaman, A. and Ryan, E. (2003) 'Reminiscing, poetry writing, and remembering boxes: Personhood-centered communication with cognitively impaired older adults.' *Activities, Adaptation & Aging 27,* 3/4, 97–112, CINAHL Plus with Full Text, EBSCO*host*, accessed on 18 June 2014.

Hammond, C. (2012) *Time Warped: Unlocking the Mysteries of Time Perception.* London: Canongate Books Ltd.

Heredia, C.G., Sage, K., Ralph, M.A L. and Berthier, M.L. (2009) 'Relearning and retention of verbal labels in a case of semantic dementia.' *Aphasiology 23,* 2, 192–209.

Hodkinson, B. (2011) 'Taking the stigma out of dementia.' *Nursing Older People 23,* 10, 8.

Hughes, J., Louw, S. and Sabat, S. (2006) 'Seeing the whole.' In J. Hughes, S. Louw and S. Sabat (eds) *Dementia: Mind, Meaning, and the Person.* e-Kindle. New York: Oxford University Press.

Innes, A. (2009) *Dementia Studies* (London edn). London: SAGE Publications Ltd.

Jaffe, I. and Benincasa, R. (2014) 'Old and Overmedicated: The Real Drug Problem in Nursing Homes.' *National Public Radio.* Available online at www.npr.org/sections/health-shots/2014/12/08/368524824/old-and-overmedicated-the-real-drug-problem-in-nursing-homes, accessed on 15 September 2015.

Jeon, Y., Govett, J., Low, L., Chenoweth, L., Fethney, J., Brodaty, H. and O'Connor, D. (2014) 'Assessment of behavioural and psychological symptoms of dementia in the era of the aged care funding instrument.' *The Internet Journal of Psychiatry 3,* 1.

Kar-Purkayastha, I. (2010) 'An epidemic of loneliness.' *The Lancet 376,* 9758, 2114–2115. Available online at www.thelancet.com/pdfs/journals/lancet/PIIS0140673610621903.pdf, accessed on 16 September 2015.

Kidd, L. (2009) *The Effect of a Poetry Writing Intervention on Self-Transcendence, Resilience, Depressive Symptoms, and Subjective Burden in Family Caregivers of Older Adults with Dementia.* ProQuest, UMI Dissertations Publishing.

Kidd, L., Zauszniewski, J. and Morris, D. (2011) 'Benefits of a poetry writing intervention for family caregivers of elders with dementia.' *Issues in Mental Health Nursing 32,* 9, 598.

King, Jr, M.L. (1963) *Letter from a Birmingham Jail.* Letter, 16 April.

Kitwood, T. (1997) *Dementia Reconsidered: The Person Comes First.* Bristol, PA: Open University Press.

Kitwood, T. and Bredin, K. (1992) 'Towards a theory of dementia care: Personhood and well-being.' *Ageing and Society 12,* 92, 269–287.

Kubler-Ross, E. (1969) *On Death and Dying.* New York, NY: Scribner.

Link, B. and Phelan, J. (2001) 'Conceptualizing stigma.' *Annual Review of Sociology 27,* 363–385.

Lipton, B. (2011) *The Biology of Belief: Unleashing the Power of Consciousness, Matter and Miracles.* London: Hay House.

Mackenzie, J. (2006) 'Stigma and dementia: East European and South Asian family carers negotiating stigma in the UK.' *Dementia 5,* 2, 233–247.

Magarey, J. (2009) *Exposure: A Journey.* Mile End, SA: Wakefield Press Pty, Limited.

Márquez, G.G. (2003) *Love in the Time of Cholera.* New York, NY: Vintage International.

Marshall, M. (2005) *Perspectives on Rehabilitation and Dementia.* London: Jessica Kingsley Publishers.

Mascher, J. (2002) 'Narrative therapy.' *Women & Therapy 25,* 2, 57–74.

Mayo Clinic (2013) *Dementia: Definition.* Available at www.mayoclinic.com/health/dementia/DS01131, acessed on 11 October 2015.

Milne, A. (2010) 'The "D" word: Reflections on the relationship between stigma, discrimination and dementia.' *Journal of Mental Health 19,* 3, 227–233.

Moore, R. (2011) Alzheimer's Australia national conference.

Mukadam, N. and Livingston, G. (2012) 'Reducing the Stigma Associated with Dementia: Approaches and Goals.' *Aging Health 8,* 4, 377.

Novotney, A. (2008) 'Finding the right words.' *Monitor 39,* 2. Available at www.apa.org/monitor/feb08/finding.aspx, accessed on 11 October 2015.

Odenheimer, G. (2006) 'Driver safety in older adults: The physician's role in assessing driving skills of older patients.' *Geriatrics 61,* 10, 14–21. In P. Gray-Vickrey (2010) 'Dementia and driving.' *Alzheimer's Care Today 11,* 3, 149–150.

Overmier, J.B. (2013) 'Learned helplessness.' *Psychology.* DOI: http://dx.doi.org/10.1093/obo/9780199828340-0112.

Payne, M. (2006) *Narrative Therapy.* London: SAGE Publications.

Pesonen, H., Remes, A. and Isola, A. (2011) 'Ethical aspects of researching subjective experiences in early-stage dementia.' *Nursing Ethics 18,* 5, 651–661.

Phillipson, L., Magee, C., Jones, S. and Skladzien, E. (2012) 'Correlates of dementia attitudes in a sample of middle-aged Australian adults.' *Australasian Journal on Ageing 33,* 3 ,158–163.

Polkinghorne, D.E. (2000) 'Narrative Therapy'. In A. E. Kazdin (ed.) *Encyclopedia of Psychology.* Washington, DC: American Psychological Association.

Powell, J. (2005) *Julie and Julia.* London: Penguin.

Rahman, S. (2014) *Living Well with Dementia: The Importance of the Person and the Environment for Wellbeing.* London: Radcliffe.

Rahman, S. (2015) *Living Better with Dementia: Good Practice and Innovation for the Future.* London: Jessica Kingsley Publishers.

Ryan, S. (2006) 'Stigma of dementia is "cruel and widespread".' *Irish Medical Times 40,* 39, 6.

Sabat, S. (2001) *The Experience of Alzheimer's Disease: Life Through a Tangled Veil.* Malden, MA: Blackwell.

Scheff, T. (1990) *Microsociology: Discourse, Emotion and Social Structure.* London: University of Chicago Press.

Scottish Dementia Working Group (2014) *About Us.* Available at www.sdwg.org.uk/home/about-us-sdwg, accessed on 3 April 2014.

Seligman, M. (2011) *Flourish: A Visionary New Understanding of Happiness and Well-being.* New York, NY: Free Press.

Simpson, J. and Roud, S. (2000) *Dictionary of English Folklore.* Oxford: Oxford University Press.

Sinclair, A.J., Morley, J.E. and Vellas, B. (2012) *Rehabilitation.* Chichester: John Wiley & Sons, Ltd.

Squires, A.J. and Hastings, M.B. (2002) *Rehabilitation of the Older Person: A Handbook for the Interdisciplinary Team.* Cheltenham: Nelson Thornes.

Swaffer, K. (2008) 'Dementia: My new world.' *Link Disability Magazine 17,* 4, 12–13.

Swaffer, K. (2011a) 'My unseen disappearing world.' *The Big Issue 389,* 16–19.

Swaffer, K. (2011b) 'Dementia: The Reality.' *Inquiry into Dementia, Early Diagnosis and Intervention.* Available at www.aph.gov.au/Parliamentary_Business/Committees/House_of_representatives_Committees?url=haa/dementia/subs/sub077%20-%20kate%20swaffer%20-%2005%20may%202012.pdf, accessed on 15 September 2015.

Swaffer, K. (2011c) 'Dementia.' *Creating Life with Words.* Available at http://kateswaffer.com/dementia, accessed 23 November 2015.

Swaffer, K. (2012a) 'Dementia, aged care, death and drugs.' *Creating Life with Words.* Available at www.kateswaffer.com/2012/09/05/dementia-aged-care-death-and-drugs.

Swaffer, K. (2012b) *Locked in Prison*. Available at www.kateswaffer. com/2011/12/29/locked-in-prison.

Swaffer, K. (2012c) *Love, Life, Loss: A Roller-Coaster of Poetry*. Kelbane, Richmond, SA: Graphic Print Group.

Swaffer, K. (2012d) 'You Live Until You Die.' In P. Willis and K. Leeson (eds) *Learning Life from Illness Stories*. Mt Gravatt, Qld: Post Pressed.

Swaffer, K. (2013) 'Creating life with words'; 'Dementia, aged care, death and drugs'; 'Dementia and human rights'; 'Dementia = social inequality'; 'Heading to aged care'; 'The human cattle yards for dementia and aged care'; 'Human rights, dementia and the elderly'; 'Locked in prison'. Available at www.kateswaffer.com/2013/05/02/ita-buttrose-on-dementia-and-human-rights, accessed on 27 November 2015.

Swaffer, K. (2014a) 'Dementia: Stigma, Language, and Dementia-friendly.' *Dementia 13*, 6, 709–716.

Swaffer, K. (2014b) 'Reinvesting in life is the best prescription.' *Australian Journal of Dementia Care*. Available at http://journalofdementiacare.com/ reinvesting-in-life-is-the-best-prescription, accessed 23 November 2015.

Swaffer, K. (2015) 'The power of language.' *Australian Journal of Dementia Care*. Available at http://journalofdementiacare.com/the-power-of-language, accessed 23 November 2015.

Taylor, R. (2007) *Alzheimer's from the Inside out*. Towson, MD: Health Professions Press.

Taylor, R. (2008) 'Is this the end of the beginning or the beginning of the end?' *Monitor 39*, 2, 25. Available at www.apa.org/monitor/feb08/isthistheend. aspx, accessed on 11 October 2015.

Temes, R. (1992) *Living with an Empty Chair: A Guide Through Grief*. Far hills, NJ: New Horizon Press Publishers.

Ticehurst, S. (2001) 'Is dementia a mental illness?' *Australian and New Zealand Journal of Psychiatry 35*, 716–723.

Travers, C., MacAndrew, M., Hines, .S, O'Reilly, M., Fielding, E., Beattie, E. and Brooks, D. (2015) 'The effectiveness of meaningful occupation interventions for people living with dementia in residential aged care: a systematic review protocol.' *JBI Database of Systematic Reviews & Implementation Report 13*, 4, 87–99.

Walker, R. (2012) *The Five Stages of Health*. London: Transworld Publishers.

Werner, P., Mittelman, M., Goldstein, D. and Heinik, J. (2012) 'Family stigma and caregiver burden in Alzheimer's disease.' *The Gerontologist 52*, 1, 89–97.

White, M., Morgan, A. and Dulwich Centre (2006) *Narrative Therapy with Children and Their Families*. Adelaide: Dulwich Centre Publications.

Zeilig, H. (2014) 'Gaps and spaces: Representations of dementia in contemporary British poetry.' *Dementia (London, England) 13*, 2, 160–175.